Aphasia Rehabilitation

The Impairment and its Consequences

Aphasia Rehabilitation

The Impairment and Its Consequences

Edited by

Nadine Martin, Ph.D.
Cynthia K. Thompson, Ph.D.
Linda Worrall, Ph.D.

PLURAL
PUBLISHING
INC.

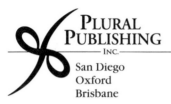

PLURAL PUBLISHING
INC.
San Diego
Oxford
Brisbane

Plural Publishing, Inc

5521 Ruffin Road
San Diego, CA 92123

e-mail: info@pluralpublishing.com
Web site: http://www.pluralpublishing.com

49 Bath Street
Abingdon, Oxfordshire OX14 1EA
United Kingdom

Typeset in 10½/13_Garamond by So Cal Graphics
Printed in the United States of America by Bang Printing

Library of Congress Cataloging-in-Publication Data
Aphasia rehabilitation : the impairment and its consequences / edited by Nadine
Martin, Cynthia K. Thompson, and Linda Worrall.
     p. ; cm.
Includes bibliographical references.
ISBN-13: 978-1-59756-162-4 (pbk.)
ISBN-10: 1-59756-162-2 (pbk.)
1. Aphasic persons--Rehabilitation--Case studies. I. Martin, Nadine, 1952- II.
Thompson, Cynthia K. III. Worrall, Linda.
[DNLM: 1. Aphasia--rehabilitation—Case Reports. WL 340.5 A6415 2007]
RC425.A665 2007
616.85'5206—dc22
                    2007036861

Contents

Preface   ix

Contributors   xiii

SECTION I   1

1   Approaches to Aphasia Treatment   3
Cynthia K. Thompson and Linda Worrall

SECTION II   25

2   A Case of Fluent Aphasia   27
Anna Basso and Audrey L. Holland

3   Treatment for Fluent Aphasia from a   31
Cognitive-Impairment Perspective
Anna Basso

4   Concentrating on the Consequences: 45
Consequence-Oriented Treatment
Audrey L. Holland

5   Impairment and Life Consequences Approaches for   63
Fluent Aphasia: Convergences and Divergences
Audrey L. Holland and Anna Basso

SECTION III   67

6   A Case of Severe Apraxia of Speech and Aphasia   69
David Howard and Nina Simmons-Mackie

7   Intervention for a Case of Severe Apraxia of Speech   75
and Aphasia: A Functional-Social Perspective
Nina Simmons-Mackie

8   Treatment for a Case of Severe Apraxia of Speech   109
and Aphasia: An Impairment-Based Perspective
David Howard

9   Impairment and Functional-Social Approaches for   125
Severe Apraxia of Speech and Aphasia: Convergences
and Divergences
Nina Simmons-Mackie and David Howard

SECTION IV   **129**

10   A Case of Nonfluent Aphasia and Agrammatism   131
Cynthia K. Thompson and Linda Worrall

11   Impairment-Based Treatment for Agrammatism from   135
a Neurolinguistic Perspective
Cynthia K. Thompson

12   Intervention for Agrammatism from a Consequences   155
Perspective
Linda Worrall

13   Impairment and Life Consequences Approaches for   171
Treatment of Nonfluent Aphasia with Agrammatism:
Convergences and Divergences
Linda Worrall and Cynthia K. Thompson

SECTION V   **175**

14   A Case of Anomic Aphasia   177
Nadine Martin and Jacqueline Hinckley

15   Intervention for Anomic Aphasia from a Functional   181
Perspective
Jacqueline Hinckley

16   Intervention for Anomic Aphasia from a Cognitive   199
Impairment-Based Perspective
Nadine Martin

17   Cognitive and Functional Interventions for Anomic   219
Aphasia: Convergences and Divergences
Jacqueline Hinckley and Nadine Martin

SECTION VI 223

18   A Case of Letter-by-Letter Reading 225
Linda J. Garcia

19   A Treatment Plan for a Letter-by-Letter Reader: 231
Intervention from an Integrated Perspective
Linda J. Garcia

SECTION VII 259

20   The State of Impairment- and Consequences-Based
Approaches to Treatment for Aphasia: Final Commentary 261
Argye Hillis, Linda Worrall, and Cynthia K. Thompson

Index 271

Preface

This book represents a meeting of minds in aphasia rehabilitation. Two approaches to aphasia rehabilitation have emerged over many years. One focuses on treating the language impairment directly, whereas the other addresses the consequences of that impairment for the individual's life. Over the past several years, advocates for each view have debated the wisdom of the other at many conferences, meetings, and in journal forums, but unfortunately, the debates have generally not resulted in a consensus approach. The lack of consensus has left practicing aphasia clinicians and people with aphasia themselves unsure about which approach is best. The chapters of this book address cases of aphasia from both viewpoints and discuss points of convergence and divergence between them. What has come from this discussion is a new awareness that, although the two approaches differ in several ways, elements of both philosophies are considered by clinicians when addressing the needs of persons with aphasia. Furthermore, the text indicates that both are necessary to address the full array of problems that people with aphasia present.

The impetus for this book began with Professor Dr. Anna Basso's book *Aphasia and Its Therapy* (Basso, 2003). In one chapter of that book, Basso expressed a need for a consensus theory of aphasia treatment, because one did not exist. Subsequently, Basso, together with Professor Dr. Audrey Holland, identified a group 15 experts in aphasia from around the world and invited them to convene for a meeting in Lerici, Italy. Nine aphasiologists participated in the first meeting, including (in alphabetical order), Anna Basso (University of Milan, Italy), Alfonso Caramazza (Harvard University, USA), Margaret Forbes (Carnegie Mellon University, USA), Linda Garcia (University of Ottawa, Canada), Nancy Helm-Estabrooks (University of North Carolina, USA), Jacqueline Hinckley (University of South Florida, USA), Audrey Holland (The University of Arizona, USA), David Howard (The University of Newcastle-on-Tyne, UK), Walter Huber (RWTH Aachen University, Germany), Nadine Martin (Temple University, USA), and Linda Worrall (The University of Queensland, Australia). Although a theory of aphasia treatment was not determined, the meeting exposed the clear differences between the philosophical bases of the impairment and consequences approaches to treatment. Some espoused an impairment approach and others a consequences approach. Hence, a second meeting was, planned to discuss the two approaches.

Those who participated in the second meeting, held in 2005, again in Lerici, Italy, were Anna Basso (University of Milan, Italy), Linda Garcia (University of Ottawa, Canada), Argye Hillis (Johns Hopkins University School of Medicine, USA), Audrey Holland (The University of Arizona, USA), David Howard (The University of Newcastle-on-Tyne, UK), Walter Huber (RWTH Aachen University, Germany), Steve Nadeau (University of Florida College of Medicine, USA), Nadine Martin (Temple University, USA), Nina Simmons-Mackie (Southeastern Louisiana University, USA), Cynthia Thompson (Northwestern University, USA),and Linda Worrall (The University of Queensland, Australia). After nearly four days of discussion, it was determined that, although there clearly are differences between the two approaches, there is likely common ground between the two. In addition, we learned that we held some beliefs that are not entirely true. For example, researchers and clinicians in the "impairment" group were unaware that their colleagues in the "consequences" group sometimes provide direct treatment for aphasic impairments. Similarly, experts in the consequences group were unaware that impairment-based professionals also sometimes directly address the functional aspects of aphasia. Furthermore, the group agreed that contention between advocates of the two approaches is not in the best interest of the profession or the clients that we treat. Therefore, we decided to tackle the problem by discussing real cases of aphasia, detailing intervention for them from both perspectives. The idea was that this process would clarify the real differences and similarities between the two approaches. We would teach each other.

Subsequent to the meeting, cases were selected. Pairs of aphasiologists, one member of the pair representing the impairment and the other representing the consequences approach, were asked to develop a treatment plan for a case allocated to them. The cases were presented at the World Federation of Neurology meeting in Buenos Aires, Argentina, in 2006. The enthusiasm and discussion generated at the meeting resulted in our writing this book.

The heart of the book presents these cases, with each addressed in one of five sections of the book. The first chapter of each section describes the case. Chapters presenting both the impairment-based and consequences approaches follow, and the final chapter in each section summarizes how the two converge and diverge. One exception is Section 6 in which both impairment and functional treatment is described by a single author.

An introductory chapter outlines the history behind each approach, conceptualizes and describes the current status of the approaches, and presents some solutions for bridging the gap between the two. The final chapter summarizes the similarities and differences between the two approaches that are captured in the pages of the book. It is concluded that both are important and should be provided for persons with aphasia and stresses that advances in our clinical training programs coupled with research evaluating the effects of both treatments, will move the profession and our science forward.

We wish to dedicate this book to Professors Anna Basso and Audrey Holland, two highly influential aphasiologists who initiated the Lerici meetings and who have significantly contributed to aphasia rehabilitation over many decades. Their influence is apparent throughout the pages of this book.

Nadine Martin, Cynthia Thompson, and Linda Worrall

Reference

Basso, A. (2003). *Aphasia and its therapy.* Oxford University Press. Oxford, UK

CONTRIBUTORS

Anna Basso, Ph.D.
Associate Professor of
Neuropsychology
University of Milan,
Milan, Italy
Chapters 2, 3, and 5

Linda Garcia, Ph.D.
Associate Professor and Chair
Audiology and Speech-Language
Pathology Program
University of Ottawa
Ottawa, Canada
Chapters 18 and 19

Argye Hillis, M.D.
Professor of Neurology and
Medicine
Department of Neurology
Johns Hopkins School of Medicine
Baltimore, Maryland
ChaPter 20

Jacqueline Hinckley, Ph.D.
Associate Professor
Department of Communication
Sciences and Disorders
University of South Florida
Tampa, Florida
Chapters 14, 15, and 17

Audrey Holland, Ph.D.
Regents' Professor Emerita
Speech and Hearing Sciences
University of Arizona
Tucson, Arizona
Chapters 2, 4, and 5

David Howard, Ph.D.
Research Development Professor
School of Education,
Communication and Language
Sciences
The University of Newcastle upon
Tyne
United Kindom
Chapters 6, 8, and 9

Nadine Martin, Ph.D.
Associate Professor
Department of Communication
Sciences and Disorders
Temple University
Phlladelphia, Pennsylvania
Chapters 14, 16, and 17

Nina Simmons-Mackie, Ph.D.
Professor and Scholar in Residence
Department of Communication
Sciences and Disorders
Southeastern Louisiana University
Hammond, Louisiana
Chapters 6, 7, and 9

Cynthia Thompson, Ph.D.
Professor
Department of Communication
Sciences and Disorders
Northwestern University
Evanston, Illinois
Chapters 1, 10, 11, 13, and 20

Linda Worrall, Ph.D.
Professor
Communications Disability Centre

School of Health and Rehabilitation
The University of Queensland
Queensland, Australia
Chapters 1, 10, 12, 13, and 20

SECTION I

1

Approaches to Aphasia Treatment

Cynthia K. Thompson and Linda Worrall

This chapter describes two approaches to aphasia treatment. The first, the "impairment-based" method, has the longest history and is therefore often considered the more traditional approach. The goal of impairment-based intervention is to provide treatment for aspects of language that are impaired. Impairment-based treatment uses models of normal language and cognitive processing to determine components and processes of the language system that have been fractionated by brain damage, and treatment is prescribed to ameliorate them. The aim of this method is to improve language ability; that is, to restore as much as possible the ability to process language. The second approach has a variety of names (functional, social, life participation, psychosocial) but all essentially target the consequences of the impairment for the person with aphasia. In this text, this approach is termed the "consequences approach." This approach uses psychosocial models to determine the impact of the aphasia on life participation, and the goal of treatment is to reduce the consequences or the impact of aphasia on a person's life. This chapter tracks the history and philosophical underpinnings of each approach and presents some distinctions, or points of disagreement between the two. Some common goals of the two approaches also are highlighted. Finally, suggestions for ways to bridge the gap be-tween the two approaches are proposed.

Impairment-Based Treatment

A Brief History

The history of impairment-focused treatment is relatively short, dating to the early 1900s. There is little mention of treatment in the literature prior to World War I, although Broca (1865) and Bas-tian (1898) discussed some rehabilitation strategies, and Gutzmann (1896), and Froeschels (1914, 1916) suggested different treatment approaches for "motor" and "sensory" aphasias. Articulation thera-py was proposed for the former; whereas, for the latter, associated with comprehension difficulty, lip reading was advocated. For both aphasia types, methods were borrowed from those used for teach-ing speech to deaf children.

Perhaps the earliest serious discussion of aphasia therapy was that published by Theodore Weisenberg and Katharine McBride (1935), in their book *Aphasia, A Clinical and Psychological Study*, which is based on a study of 60 cases of aphasia. Dr. Weisenberg, then a Professor of Neurology and Dr. McBride a psychologist, both at the University of Pennsylvania, undertook their study of apha-sia primarily to describe the "mental changes" present in aphasia. In addition, they examined the effects of treating, or more precise-ly "reeducating" the aphasic patients that they studied. Due to a lack of valid tests for aphasia at the time, part of the work also in-volved developing behavioral assessment tools to document "men-tal changes" and the effects of treatment.[1] The principles of treat-ment were to: (a) adapt training to the individual patient, so as to deal with his or her particular deficits, and (b) take advantage of the patient's retained abilities. A medical model was employed: rather than prescribing treatment based on the type of aphasia, each case was considered a clinical problem, which required "careful and

---

[1]Weisenberg points out that the study was initiated based on a serendipitous finding: two of his graduate students in neuropsychiatry administered Henry Head's tests for aphasia to the other students in the program. Surprisingly, the students' performed similarly to Head's aphasic patients!

continuous study, and training especially adapted to overcome specific deficits and make the most of abilities which [were] still within the patient's power" (p. 383). Interestingly, another important principle of treatment concerned psychosocial issues: (c) "to increase the interest and value of the practice by connecting it with daily experience" (p. 388). In addition, Weisenberg and McBride suggested that "a very important and sometimes the most important function of the reeducation is to contribute to the patient's sense of well-being and to increase his morale" (p. 391). Based on extensive testing, training was focused on specific abilities, including production of various speech sounds, writing letter forms, producing and writing words, and comprehending and producing sentence structure, using primarily drilling exercises.

During and following World War II treatment for aphasia became more common, influenced by the need to treat war-wounded patients with head injuries. In this period Soviet neurologists developed a system of rehabilitation hospitals, which provided "the ordinary surgical, pharmacological and physiotherapeutic methods of treatment . . . supplemented by active exercises, occupational therapy and speech re-education" (Luria, 1963, p. ix). Similarly, in America, Veterans Administration hospitals became the venue for treating these patients. Treatment continued to focus on the language impairment using various methods.

A. R. Luria, a Russian neurologist and psychologist, worked under the premise that higher cognitive functions are supported by an "integral system of . . . cortical areas, working in close collaboration with each other." He further noted that if "one of the cortical areas subserving a given function is destroyed, the system can be re-organized in such a manner as to secure continuation of the activity in question by other means, involving the participation of other, intact areas of the brain" (p. xiii). He supported the idea that treatment has a direct effect on the brain, that it can be reorganized to support impaired "functions" such as speech, writing, or reading. Importantly, a major premise of successful treatment was that a well-defined theoretical basis for it "is absolutely essential if the re-training is to be successful" (p.135). Thus, intervention methods proposed by Luria aimed to influence the various brain links that support restoration of the impaired function. "The aim of such retraining is to reconstruct the functional system" (p. 138). Methods used by Luria exploited the rules of normal grammar, for example, the fact that all sentences must have a predicate, and methods sought to "re-teach" language focused on these rules. The idea was to decompose what was once automatic, for example, sentence production, into component rules, to explicitly teach these rules, to have the patient practice them repeatedly, and to thereby restore them to automatic usage. Luria suggested that "profound reconstruction [results from] transfer of speech to the level of conscious action, [followed by] subsequent automatization" (p. 154).

American clinicians also espoused an impairment-based approach during the post-World War II period. Again evaluation of the patient revealed deficit patterns and treatment was designed based on the theoretical position of the clinician. Hildred Schuell, a prominent clinician of the time, believed that aphasia is a unitary disorder; that is, she believed that there is only one aphasia and all aphasias are the same, but that other concomitant visual, sensorim-otor, or other impairments confounded the deficit, resulting in several different deficit patterns (Schuell, Jenkins, & Jimenez-Pabon, 1964). She also espoused that the auditory modality played a central role in the aphasia and recovery from it; thus, she prescribed intensive, repetitive auditory stimulation for all patients, and based on the constellation of individual deficits, stimulation was provided in other impaired modalities as well (Schuell, Carroll, & Street, 1955). Joseph Wepman, another leading figure, agreed that there is only one aphasia; however, he suggested that aphasia is a thought-centered problem (Wepman, 1951). Thus, treatment too was thought-centered. That is, treatment was aimed at the content of what was to be communicated using three treatment principles: stimulation, facilitation, and motivation. Stimulation was provided only when the patient was motivated, and a response relaying a thought was facilitated, without regard to its form. These approaches were considered holistic, termed stimulation-facilitation methods. Rather than focusing on the structure of language, that is, retraining linguistic rules as prescribed by Luria, nonspecific stimulation was used to facilitate general language recovery.

Stimulation-facilitation type treatment remained the primary approach for aphasia treatment until the 1960s and 1970s. Among the events that moved aphasia treatment forward was Norman Geshwind's classic paper: "Dissconnection Syndromes in Animals and Man" (Geschwind, 1965), which renewed interest in the relation between the brain and language. Subsequently, the aphasia syndromes were redescribed using more detailed linguistic analyses and more sophisticated anatomical models (Goodglass & Kaplan, 1972) and, rather than using the same treatment for all, treatment for specific aphasic impairments were developed.

Contemporary Impairment Treatment

The practice of impairment-based treatment for aphasia has continued to change and grow in the past few decades. This growth was influenced by scientific advances in several areas, including cognitive neuroscience, neuroscience, psycholinguistics, neurolinguistics, cognitive neuropsychology, and treatment research findings. In the domain of cognitive neuroscience, neuroimaging studies showed that many early ideas about the brain and language were not completely correct. The most profound finding was that language is subserved by a highly interactive neural network, which includes parts of the brain that were not previously identified as language regions such as the fusiform gyrus and the inferior temporal region. We also learned that the classic language areas are involved in aspects of language processing that were not previously identified. For example, neuroimaging studies with healthy volunteers showed that Broca's area is involved in phonological, semantic, and morphosyntactic processing (Ben-Shachar, Hendler, Kahy, Ben-Bashat, et al., 2003; Sonty, Mesulam, Thompson, Johnson et al., 2003, and many others). We learned that the classic aphasia syndromes do not coincide with specific brain lesions and that the deficit patterns that many patients present do not coincide with the behavioral patterns of the classic aphasias. For example, Broca's aphasia does not result from lesions in Broca's area alone; most lesions are much more widespread, often extending to the prefrontal, motor, sensory, and even parietal-temporal regions (Vanier & Caplan, 1990). Furthermore, these patients often show comprehension, in addition to production, deficits.

Neuroscience research also impacted our thinking about the neural mechanisms of recovery and the role of the environment in shaping recovery. Results of animal studies showed that motor learning, tactile, and auditory stimulation affect organization of the primary motor, somatosensory, and auditory cortices, respectively (Greenough, Larson, & Withers, 1985; Recanzone, Schreiner, & Merzenich, 1993; Van Praag, Kempermann, & Gage, 1999). Studies of rehabilitative training after brain injury also showed that the brain has the capacity to reorganize (Nudo, Milliken, Jenkins, & Merzenich, 1996; Xerri, Merzenich, Peterson, & Jenkins, 1998), indicating that experience directly shapes physiological reorganization following brain damage. Several studies examining training-induced recovery from aphasia also indicated that treatment affects the neural networks engaged to support language (see Thompson, 2005, for review).

Psycholinguistic research also impacted our thinking about aphasia and treatment for it. For example, in the 1980s, in the domain of sentence processing, researchers began testing patient's ability to process complex sentences using experimental paradigms such as cross-modal priming (Swinney, & Zurif, 1995; Zurif, Swinney, Prather, Solomon, & Bushell, 1993). The results indicated that on-line processing performance may differ from off-line performance. For example, both Broca's and Wernicke's aphasic patients showed difficulty comprehending complex sentences using traditional off-line sentence-picture matching tasks. However, Wernicke's, but not Broca's patients evinced normal on-line processing ability. Although these findings have been challenged (Blumstein, Byma, Kurowski, Hourihan, Brown, & Hutchinson, 1998; Dickey, Choy, & Thompson, 2007), this work led to a better understanding of the processing mechanisms underlying sentence comprehension. Neurolinguistic theories of aphasia also advanced our work. For example, the Trace Deletion Hypothesis and its variants suggested particular deficiencies in sentence comprehension and strategies used by aphasic patients to overcome them (Grodzinsky 1990). These, and other, findings concerning patient's ability to map thematic roles onto sentence forms (Linebarger, Schwartz, & Saffran, 1993) impacted treatments for sentence deficits in aphasia. Thompson and colleagues used these theories and data to develop treatment for sentence comprehension and production deficits associated with agrammatism (see Thompson, Chapter 11, this volume).

In the 1980s, the discipline of cognitive neuropsychology was developed (Coltheart, 1984). One purpose of the discipline was to build models of normal cognitive processing, for example, models of lexical processing and sentence production, using data derived from brain-damaged patients. These models had significant impact on intervention for aphasia, both in terms of testing for patient deficits and guiding treatment for them. Chapters by Basso,

Howard, and Martin (this volume) used this approach for treating patients with fluent aphasia, severe apraxia of speech and aphasia, and anomic aphasia, respectively.

In the past few decades there also has been an increase in research examining the effects of treatment. Early treatment efficacy work used groups of aphasic patients to determine the general outcomes of treatment (see for example, Basso, Capitani, & Vignolo, 1979; Wertz, Collins, Weiss, Kurtzke et al., 1981). Although this work showed that impairment-based treatment does, in fact, improve language ability in aphasia, more recent work has sought to examine the effects of specific treatment for specific language deficits. Much of this work has used single subject controlled experimental analysis to detail patterns of recovery in individual patients (see Thompson 2006, for review), with results showing that treatment focused explicitly on language deficits results in improvement. Studies have shown that generalization to untrained structures often is forthcoming, and in addition, that changes in spontaneous language also results. In particular, treatments guided by models and theories of normal language representation and processing, as well as psycholinguistic and neurolinguistic research findings, have been shown to be most successful.

Some Premises of Impairment-Based Treatment

One of the primary premises of impairment-based treatment is that the normal language system is fractionated in aphasia. This notion is based on the fact that some, but not all, domains of language are impaired in aphasia and that variations in the components of language that are impaired are common. For example, some patients have primary deficits in naming, but naming of nouns may be more impaired than verbs, and when the naming deficit is carefully analyzed, the underlying source of the deficit may differ across patients. Some may show deficits in semantic aspects of naming; others may have difficulty accessing the phonological form of words. The impairment-based approach seriously considers such deficit patterns and treatment is guided by what is known about normal language processing. In addition, impairment-based approaches hold that language is not lost. Rather the problem lies in access to language or the ability to engage the required processing routines to compute language. Thus, as pointed out by Basso in Chapter 5, the aim of treatment is to "help the patient to reclaim as much as possible of the underlying damaged capacity to process language in the same way as a "normal" person processes language".

Another premise of impairment-based approaches to aphasia treatment is that functional language use will emerge as a by-product of successful treatment. Thus, the ability to participate in communication activities will result from treatment. However, intervention requires ongoing assessment of the impact of treatment on functional language. Thus, although predictions can be made about learning and generalization, nothing is assumed. If generalization does not result, the focus of the treatment is altered; it is either shifted to different structures/impairments and/or focused directly on language use in daily activities. Indeed, generalization to untrained language and to functional communication contexts is the gold standard of aphasia treatment; without it treatment may be deemed ineffective.

The Consequences Approach

The purpose of this section is to introduce readers to the concepts and principles of consequences-focused aphasia rehabilitation. A brief history of the approach introducing some of the terms used is followed by a summary of the main influences that have shaped the approach. Finally, some of the main principles and values that underlie the approach are described.

This is the first known occasion that the term "consequences-focused approach" has been used and this construct is a combination of several terms used in the literature. In an effort to make this information accessible to readers unfamiliar with the terminology and constructs of a consequences-focused approach, the reader is referred to more detailed discussions of specific approaches throughout this introductory chapter.

Speech-language pathologists have long recognized that aphasia has a significant impact on people's lives. The disability associated with aphasia is characterized by decreased quality of life (Ross & Wertz, 2003), increased prevalence of depression (Code & Herrman, 2003), and social isolation (Hirsch & Holland, 2000). As Parr, Byng, Gilpin, and Ireland (1997) note, language is the currency of relationships; therefore, aphasia has a widespread effect on partners, children, parents, siblings, friends; and colleagues; and hence it has broader effects in the community.

Martha Taylor Sarno began the recorded history of the Functional Communication Profile (FCP; Sarno, 1969). Audrey Holland's Communicative Abilities in Daily Living (CADL; Holland, 1980) and other measures emerged later. Much of the early literature drew heavily from the rehabilitation approach by publishing the Functional Communication Pion literature and the theoretical frameworks of pragmatics (see Holland and Hinckley, 2002 for a brief history of the influence of pragmatics). Since that time, there has been an exponential increase in the literature surrounding the consequences approach.

In the modern era of the consequences approach, three major influences external to speech-language pathology have changed the way it is now perceived and valued within speech-language pathology. The first of these was the widespread influence and acceptance of disability models such as the World Health Organization's International Classification of Functioning, Disability, and Health (ICF; WHO, 2001). The earliest version of the ICF (then titled International Classification on Impairments, Disabilities and Handicaps) appeared in 1980 and the latest version was endorsed by the World Health Organization in 2001. The second external influence has been a greater demand by health care payers for increased accountability for their rehabilitation dollar (Frattali, 1992) and the consequential interest in functional outcome measurement (Frattali, 1998). Finally, and more recently, a greater voice has been given to people with disabilities themselves. Accordingly, the disability movement has focused attention away from the person with the disability to the disabling society in which they live. This approach has been labeled the social approach and as a consequence, legislation now exists in many countries that prohibits discrimination against people with disabilities (see Byng and Duchan, 2005; Jordan and Kaiser, 1996). Client-focused rehabilitation (e.g., Cott, Teare, McGilton, & Lineker, 2006; Worrall, 2006) is an off-shoot of the disability movement which places more power for decision-making in the client's hands. This process is not so much about a different therapy, but a different way of deciding what therapy is to be provided.

Each of these three main influences is now described in more detail and their specific application to aphasia rehabilitation outlined. Through this discussion, the major features of the consequences-focused approach are illuminated.

The Influence of Models of Disability

Although there are various models of disability (see Frattali, 1998 for a review), the World Health Organization's (WHO) conceptual framework has emerged as the most widely accepted internationally. The most recent WHO conceptual framework, the International Classification of Functioning, Disability and Health (ICF, WHO 2001) was heavily influenced by the Canadian based Disability Creation Process (Fougeyrollas, Noreau, Bergeron, Cloutier, Dion, & St-Michel, 1998).

The conceptual framework of the ICF is shown in Figure 1–1 and the terminology is shown in Table 1-1. As the overall aim of the ICF, like the International Classification of Diseases (ICD) and others in the family of WHO classifications is to provide a universal language, it is important that the correct terminology be used and Table 1-1 demonstrates the correct use of terms. Kagan, Simmons-Mackie, Rowland, Huijbregts, Shumway, McEwen, et al. (2007) translated the ICF into a framework (A-FROM) for measuring real-life outcomes in aphasia. During this process they simplified the concepts in the ICF and used terminology relevant for people concerned with aphasia.

The consequences approach could be interpreted as targeting outcomes in the Participation component of the ICF. Hence, aphasia therapy can target the Participation dimension directly or indirectly through Activities and the Contextual Factors, whether they be external to the person (Environmental Factors) or internal (Personal Factors). Working at the impairment level to gain greater participation is also considered to be within the scope of this approach, but it is not the main or even sole approach. The ICF is not a linear model; hence, by implication, there is no assumption that the process of rehabilitation should start with targeting the impairment and then moving on to "functional" outcomes or vice versa. The arrows in Figure 1–1 indicate that the components are multidirectional and clearly influence each other. By implication, this means that aphasia therapy may directly target the environment, for example, and this may in turn affect Participation or even the Impairment. The ICF, therefore,

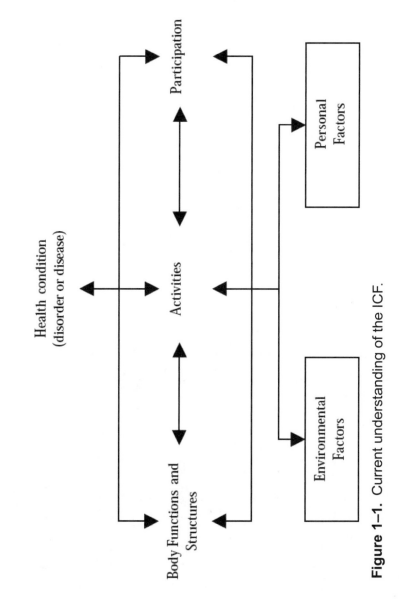

Figure 1–1. Current understanding of the ICF.

13

Table 1–1. Overview of ICF

	Part 1: Functioning and Disability		Part 2: Contextual Factors	
Components	Body Functions and Structures	Activities and Participation	Environmental Factors	Personal Factors
Domains	Body functions and structures	Life areas (tasks, actions)	External influences on functioning and disability	Internal influences on functioning and disability
Constructs	Change in body functions (physiological) Change in body structures (anatomic)	Capacity executing tasks in a standard environment Performance executing tasks in the current environment	Facilitating or hindering impact of features of the physical, social, and attitudinal world	Impact of attributes of the person

challenges the traditional belief that aphasia therapy must begin by treating the impairments of language and then seek to generalize these to everyday life. The consequences approach might target any of the nonimpairment ICF components directly or indirectly. Basso (2003) describes the consequences or functional approach as "top down," meaning that Participation is the primary goal and therefore is targeted first and foremost. This contrasts with a "bottom up" approach in which the components of language are targeted first and then generalized to the broader domain of Participation.

There have been many publications that have interpreted aphasia and its consequences within the ICF with the most recent surrounding a debate about assessment in aphasia using the ICF (see Forum led by Ross and Wertz, 2005). Similarly, there is a developing research base that has examined the application of the ICF to aphasia. The research has attempted to define the everyday communication activities in which people with aphasia engage for the Activities/Participation component of the ICF (Worrall, McCooey, Davidson, Larkins, & Hickson, 2002), the Environmental Factors that either hinder or help people with aphasia in the community (Howe, Worrall, & Hickson, in press) and the relationships between the ICF dimensions and quality of life (Cruice, Worrall, Hickson, & Murison, 2003)

In summary, the consequences approach has been influenced by models of disability and the approach has been described in terms of the ICF. The consequences approach may directly or indirectly target Activity/Participation, Environmental Factors, or Personal Factors. Within aphasia, these are described as the everyday communication activities such as conversations, telephoning, completing forms, and participating in work or educational roles (Activity/Participation), other people's communicative accommodation to a person with aphasia or their attitude to a person with aphasia (Environmental Factors), or the existing resilience, coping skills, optimism, identity, age, or culture of a person with aphasia (Personal Factors).

The Influence of Increased Accountability

In her seminal article, Frattali (1992) highlighted the link between increased accountability in health care systems and functional communication outcomes. In this article, she argued that payers expect significant practical improvements on functional goals. In a later text, she urged speech-language pathologists to "listen and respond to the softest voices"—the consumers of speech-language pathology services. She predicted that the next change in health care would be one of displacement of power where consumers take the lead. In response to this consumer-driven accountability, Worrall (2006) reviewed existing evidence about the goals of people with aphasia as a window for determining what approach to therapy people with aphasia may want. Although many goals crossed the biopsychosocial spectrum, there was much emphasis on goals such as participation in life activities, relationships, and personal self-esteem. There has yet to be a rigorous study about how the goals of people with aphasia may change over time or the goals of family members who have also been affected by aphasia.

Calls for increased accountability, in the form of outcome measurement, prompted speech-language pathologists to focus on defining and measuring functional communication outcomes in aphasia. Managed care in countries such as the United States also focused therapists' attention on achieving functional outcomes effectively and efficiently.

The Influence of the Disability Movement/Social Model

The third influence on aphasia rehabilitation that has prompted the development of the consequences approach has stemmed from a greater voice by consumers. The disability movement has been influential in legislation and policy and has created a greater awareness of the perspectives and priorities of people with disability. The disability movement and the social model of practice that it promotes, identifies a disabling society as the source of their disability, rather than the impairment itself. Although this concept has influenced health care and society more generally, it has also instigated subtle changes in rehabilitation practice. The social model philosophy suggests that the efforts of speech-language pathology should be predominantly directed at the disabling society (external to the person with aphasia) and, hence, there has been a need to define "accessibility" for people with aphasia (see Bunning & Horton, 2007 or Worrall, Rose, Howe, McKenna, & Hickson, 2007). Aphasia-friendly environments have, therefore, become another focus in the consequences approach.

It is unlikely that the literature of the disability movement accurately reflects the views of people with an acquired communication disability such as aphasia. They have traditionally not been vocal consumers; however, the views of people with aphasia are beginning to be heard and are helping to define accessibility for communication disabilities. In this way, they are contributing to and shaping the focus of the modern day "consequences approach."

In summary, the catalysts for the consequences approach go some way to defining and describing the approach, but there have also been several attempts to define the approach and establish some core principles. Worrall (2000a) reviews the definitions of functional communication and concludes that no definition can capture the multidimensional and individualized nature of the concept. The definition of functional communication assessment however as "the ability of an individual to communicate in his or her own everyday environment" (Worrall, 1995) may still be relevant. Byng and Duchan (2005) extracted principles of aphasia therapy from the social model philosophy. They are: equalising social relations, creating authentic involvement, creating engaging experiences, establishing user control, and becoming accountable to users. They point out that the social model is not a therapy approach in itself and can be applied to impairment-based therapies as well as other forms of intervention.

Similarly, the Life Participation Approach in Aphasia (LPAA, 2001) describes some basic principles for the management of aphasia. These are: (1) the explicit goal of intervention is enhancement of life participation, (2) all those affected are entitled to services, (3) measures of success include documented life enhancement, (4) both personal and environmental factors are targets of intervention, and (5) emphasis is on availability of services as needed at all stages.

Worrall (2000b) suggested that professional values are important to practicing a consequences approach. These include the values associated with shared decision-making, individualization, social justice, the strengths perspective, and accountability. Byng, Cairns, and Duchan (2002) take this one step further and suggest that speech-language pathologists' dissatisfaction with their roles as aphasia therapists are attributable to a mismatch between personal and organizational values. They then describe the values of Connect, the communication disability network established in the United Kingdom and how a values-based approach may lead to increased satisfaction with service provision to people with aphasia.

The above statements of values and principles of a consequences approach to aphasia therapy may not distinguish it from impairment-based approaches. The influences, principles, and values of the consequences approach are, however, at the heart of the approach. In the same way that models of language processing or brain function have influenced impairment-based therapy, models of disability (the ICF in particular) are guiding therapy that focuses on the consequences of aphasia. In the same way that there are a multitude of therapy tasks that can be used in impairment-based therapy, there are also many therapy tasks that can be used in therapy targeting the consequences of aphasia. Some of these tasks may even be the same. However, a therapist who consciously practices a consequences-focussed approach will fully understand the influences that have shaped the approach and will be practicing from core principles and values that have shaped the approach.

Differences and Similarities
Between the Two Approaches

The discussions above highlight crucial differences between impairment and functional approaches to aphasia treatment. There are clear philosophical differences, which influence the targets of intervention at least to some extent. Impairment treatment operates on the view that aphasia is a language impairment; thus treatment is focused on language. Conversely, consequences-based treatment is based on the idea that aphasia is a psychosocial disorder, both language and communication abilities are impaired; thus, barriers that preclude use of these abilities in life become the focus of intervention. In fact, aphasia is both an impairment disorder and a functional disorder. The term "aphasia" originated from the Greek work "aphatos" meaning "speechless," which derived from "phanai", meaning "speak"; and the definition of aphasia is that it is a partial or total inability to produce and understand speech as a result of brain damage. Aphasia is also, undeniably, a psychosocial deficit. Clearly, the inability to produce or understand language affects the life participation of persons with aphasia. Interpersonal relationships, participation in social and other events, and employability, among other factors, are affected.

There are also some similarities between the two approaches, and the chapters in this book highlight them. One similarity is that the overarching goal of both methods is to help people with aphasia communicate as affectively as possible in the environment. Advocates of both approaches also agree that treatment should be accessible to all persons with aphasia, regardless of time poststroke. Finally, there is some overlap in the treatment methods used.

Bridging the Gap Between Impairment- and Consequence-Oriented Approaches

Bridging the gap between impairment- and consequence-based approaches is necessary to address the full constellation of problems that aphasic people present. As pointed out by Hillis, Worrall, and Thompson in Chapter 20, "continuing to debate about which approach is better is not in the best interest of persons with aphasia or his or her family members, nor does this foster a positive professional image for our clients, students, or colleagues in related fields." The chapters in this book highlight the importance of both approaches and we hope that they will help to change our attitudes and our thinking about what comprises optimal treatment. Indeed, it appears that both approaches can and should be used with persons with aphasia.

One question that has confronted clinicians and researchers in aphasia is whether or not it is within the purview of speech-language pathologists to treat the psychosocial aspects of aphasia. As noted above, although traditional aphasia treatment focused on language impairments, it also is concerned with the consequences of aphasia. Weisenberg and McBride (1935) and other early advocates of impairment-based aphasia treatment expressed the need to consider the functional aspects of aphasia. Until recently, however, explicit methods for doing this were not available. The life participation approaches discussed in the chapters in this book provide these methods. Because the field of communication sciences and disorders is about communication, we suggest that speech-language pathologists should be the providers of both impairment and consequence-based intervention.

The future of aphasia treatment is exciting. Imagine a situation in which all aphasia therapists were equipped to draw from a wide range of techniques to meet each individual patient's goals. This would require not only changes in our attitudes about treatment, but also changes in the way that we train clinicians in academic programs. What is clear is that if the two approaches are to be used, clinicians must be trained in both.

Another mechanism that will undoubtedly serve to bridge the gap is continued research investigating the effects of both impairment and consequence-based treatments. Our data, not our word, will engender confidence in the approaches that we take and will eliminate questions now, and in the future, about their value.

Summary

This chapter reviewed impairment and consequence-based approaches to aphasia treatment from a historical perspective and highlighted differences between them. We also addressed some common ground shared by both. What follows in this book are examples of each approach that we hope will serve to foster a better understanding of the two methods and serve as a catalyst for bringing the two together. Changes in attitudes of clinicians and researchers about the two approaches will help to dilute the gap that presently exists between them. An understanding that provision of both is essential to foster maximal recovery is required. Educating aphasia clinicians in both methods, and encouraging their use and integration also are needed. Finally, continued empirical evaluations of the effects of treatment will help bridge the gap between them.

References

Basso, A. (2003). *Aphasia and its therapy.* Oxford, UK: Oxford University Press.

Basso, A., Capitani, E., & Vignolo, L. A. (1979). Influence of rehabilitation of language skills in aphasic patients: A controlled study. *Archives of Neurology, 36,* 190–196.

Bastian, H. C. (1898). *A treatise on aphasia and other speech defects.* London: Lewis.

Ben-Shachar, M., Hendler, T., Kahn, I., Ben-Bashat, D., & Grodzinsky, Y. (2003). The neural reality of syntactic transformations: Evidence from functional magnetic resonance imaging. *Psychological Science, 14,* 433–440.

Blumstein, S., Byma, G., Kurowski, K., Hourihan, J., Brown, T., & Hutchinson, A. (1998). On-line processing of filler-gap constructions in aphasia. *Brain and Language, 61,* 149–168.

Broca, P. P. (1865). Sur le siege de la faculte du language articule. *Bulletin d'Anthropologie, 6,* 377–393.

Bunning, K., & Horton, S. (2007). "Border crossing" as a route to inclusion: A shared cause with people with a learning disability? *Aphasiology, 21*(1), 9–22

Byng, S., Cairns, D., & Duchan, J. (2002). Values in practice and practising values. *Journal of Communication Disorders, 35,* 89–106.

Byng, S., & Duchan, J. (2005). Social model philosophies and principles: Their applications to therapies for aphasia. *Aphasiology, 19*(10–11), 906–922.

Code, C., & Herrmann, M. (2003). The relevance of emotional and psychosocial factors in aphasia to rehabilitation *Neuropsychological Rehabilitation, 13*(1/2), 109–132.

Coltheart, M. (1984). Editorial. *Cognitive Neuropsychology, 1,* 1–8.

Cott, C. A., Teare, G., McGilton, K. S., & Lineker, S. (2006). Reliability and construct validity of the Client-Centred Rehabilitation Questionnaire. *Disability and Rehabilitation, 28*(22), 1387–1397.

Cruice, M., Worrall, L., Hickson, L., & Murison, R. (2003). Finding a focus for quality of life with aphasia: social and emotional health, and psychological well-being. *Aphasiology, 17*(4), 333–353.

Dickey, M. W., Choy, J., & Thompson, C. K. (2007). Real-time comprehension of wh-movement in aphasia: Evidence from eyetracking while listening. *Brain and Language, 100,* 1–22.

Forum. (2005). *Aphasiology, 19*(9), 860–900.

Fougeyrollas, P., Noreau, L., Bergeron, H., Cloutier, R., Dion, S., & St-Michel, G. (1998). Social consequences of long term impairments and disabilities: Conceptual approach and assessment of handicap. *International Journal of Rehabilitation Research, 21*(2), 127–141.

Frattali, C. M. (1992). Functional assessment of aphasia: Merging public policy with clinical views. *Aphasiology, 6,* 63–83.

Frattali, C. M. (1998). *Measuring outcomes in speech-language pathology.* New York: Thieme.

Froeschels, E. (1914). Ueber die behandlung der aphasien. *Archiv fur Psychiatrie und Nervenkrankheiten, 53,* 221–261.

Froeschels, E. (1916). Zur behandlung der motorischen aphasie. *Archiv fur Psychiatrie und Nervenkrankheiten, 56,* 1–19.

Geschwind, N. (1965). Disconnection syndromes in animals and man. *Brain, 88,* 237-294.

Goodglass, H., & Kaplan, E. (1972). *The assessment of aphasia and related disorders.* Philadelphia: Lea and Febiger.

Greenough, W., Larson, J., & Withers, G. (1985). Effects of unilateral and bilateral training in a reaching task on dendritic branching of neurons in the rat motor sensory forelimb cortex. *Behavioral Neural Biology, 44,* 301-314.

Grodzinsky, Y. (1990). *Theoretical perspectives on language deficits.* Cambridge, MA: MIT Press.

Gutzmann, H. (1896). Heilungsversuche bei centromotorischer und centrosensoricher Aphasie. *Archiv fur Psychiatrie und Nervenkrankheiten, 28,* 354-378.

Hirsch, F., & Holland, A. (2000). Beyond activity: Measuring participation in society and quality of life. In L. Worrall & C. Frattali (Eds.), *Neurogenic communication disorders: A functional approach* (pp. 35-54). New York: Thieme.

Holland, A. L. (1980). *Communicative Abilities in Daily Living.* Baltimore, MD: University Park Press.

Holland, A. L., & Hinckley, J. J. (2002). Assessment and treatment of pragmatic aspects of communication in aphasia. In A. Hillis (Ed.) *Handbook of adult language disorders: Integrating cognitive neuropsychology, neurology and rehabilitation.* Philadelphia: Psychology Press.

Howe, T. Worrall, L. E. Hickson, L. M. (in press). Observing people with aphasia: Environmental factors that influence their community participation. *Aphasiology.*

Jordan, L., & Kaiser, W. (1996). *Aphasia: A social approach.* London: Chapman and Hal.

Kagan, A., Simmons-Mackie, N., Rowland, A., Huijbregts, M., Shumway, E., McEwen, S., et al. (2007). Counting what counts: A framework for capturing real-life outcomes of aphasia intervention. *Aphasiology,* 1-23.

Linebarger, M., Schwartz, M. F., & Saffran, E. (1983). Sensitivity to grammatical structure in so-called agrammatic aphasics. *Cognition, 13,* 361-392.

LPAA Project Group. (2001). Life Participation Approach to Aphasia: A statement of values for the future. In R. Chapey (Ed.), *Language intervention strategies in aphasia and related neurogenic communication disorders* (4th ed., pp. 235-245). Philadelphia: Lippincott, Williams & Wilkins.

Luria, A. R. (1963). *Restoration of function after brain injury.* Oxford, UK: Pergamon Press.

Nudo, R., Milliken, G., Jenkins, W., & Merzenich, M. (1996). Neural substrates for the effects of rehabilitate training on motor recovery after ischemic infarct. *Science, 171,* 1791-1794.

Parr, S., Byng, S., Gilpin, S., & Ireland, C. (1997). *Talking about aphasia: Living with loss of language after stroke.* Buckingham: Open University Press.

Recanzone, G., Schreiner, C., & Merzenich, M. (1993). Plasticity in the frequency representation of the primary auditory cortex following discrimination training in adult owl monkeys. *Journal of Neuroscience, 13,* 87–103.

Ross, K. B., & Wertz, R. T. (2003). Quality of life with and without aphasia. *Aphasiology, 17,* 355–364.

Sarno, M. T. (1969). *The functional communication profile: Manual of directions.* New York: Institute of Rehabilitation Medicine.

Schuell, H., Carroll, V., & Street, B. (1955). Clinical treatment of aphasia. *Journal of Speech and Hearing Disorders, 20,* 43–53.

Schuell, H., Jenkins, J. J., & Jimenez-Pabon, E. (1964). *Aphasia in adults.* New York: Harper & Row.

Sonty, S. P., Mesulam, M-M, Thompson, C.K., Johnson, N. A., Weintraub, S., Parrish, T.B., Gitelman, D.R. (2003). Primary Progressive Aphasia: PPA and the language network. *Annals of Neurology, 53*(1), 35–49.

Sparks, R., Helm, N., & Albert, M. (1974). Aphasia rehabilitation resulting from Melodic Intonation Therapy. *Cortex, 10,* 303–316.

Swinney, D., & Zurif, E. (1995). Syntactic processing in aphasia. *Brain and Language, 50,* 225–239.

Thompson, C. K. (2005). Plasticity of language networks. In M. Baudry, X. Bi, & S. S. Schrieber (Eds.). *Syntaptic plasticity: Basic mechanisms to clinical applications* (pp. 343–355). New York: Marcel Dekker, Inc.

Thompson, C. K. (2006). Single subject controlled experiments in aphasia: The science and the state of the science. *Journal of Communication Disorders, 39,* 266–291.

Vanier, M. & Caplan, D. (1990). CT-scan correlates of agrammatism. In L. Menn & L. Obler (Eds.), *Agrammatic aphasia: A cross-language narrative sourcebook* (pp. 37–114). Amsterdam/Philadelphia: John Benjamins.

Van Praag, H., Kempermann, G., & Gage, F. (1999). Running increases cell proliferation and neurogenesis in the adult mouse dentate gyrus. *Nature Neuroscience, 2,* 266–270.

Weisenberg, T. H., & McBride, K. E. (1935). *Aphasia: A clinical and psychological study.* New York: The Commonwealth Fund.

Wepman, J. M. (1951). *Recovery from aphasia.* New York: Ronald Press.

Wertz, R. T., Collins, M. J., Weiss, D., Kurtzke, J. E., Friden, T., Brookshire, R. H., Pierce, J., Holzapple, P., Hubbaard, D. J., Porch, B. E., West, J. A., Davis, L., Matovitch, V., Morley, G. K., & Resurreccion, E. (1981). Verterans Administration cooperative study on aphasia: A comparison of individual and group treatment. *Journal of Speech and Hearing Disorders, 24,* 580–594.

Wilson, I. B., & Cleary, P. D. (1995). Linking clinical variables with health-related quality of life. *Journal of American Medical Association, 273,* 59–68.

World Health Organization (WHO). (2001) *International Classification of Functioning, Disability and Health (ICF)*. Geneva, Switzerland: Author.

Worrall, L. (1995). The functional communication perspective In D. Muller & C. Code (Eds.), *Treatment of aphasia* (pp. 47–69). London: Whurr Publishers.

Worrall, L. (2000a). A conceptual framework for a functional approach to acquired neurogenic disorders of communication and swallowing. In L. Worrall & C. Frattali (Eds.), *Neurogenic communication disorders: A functional approach* (pp. 3–18). New York: Thieme.

Worrall, L. (2000b). The influence of professional values on the functional communication approach in aphasia. In L. Worrall & C. Frattali (Eds.), *Neurogenic communication disorders: A functional approach* (pp. 191–205). New York: Thieme.

Worrall, L. (2006). Professionalism and functional outcomes. *Journal of Communication Disorders, 3,* 320–327.

Worrall, L., McCooey, R., Davidson, B., Larkins, B., & Hickson, L. (2002). The validity of functional assessments of communication and the Activity/Participation components of the ICIDH-2: Do they reflect what really happens in real-life? *Journal of Communication Disorders, 35*(2), 107–137.

Worrall, L., Rose, T., Howe, T., McKenna, K., & Hickson, L. (2007). Developing an evidence-base for communication accessibility for people with aphasia *Aphasiology, 21*(1), 124–136.

Xerri, C., Merzenich, M., Peterson, B., & Jenkins, W. (1998). Plasticity of primary somatosensory cortex paralleling sensorimotor skill recovery from stroke in adult monkeys. *Journal of Neurophysiology, 79,* 2119–2148.

Zurif, E., Swinney, D., Prather, P., Solomon, J., & Bushell, C. (1993). On-line analysis of syntactic processing in Broca's and Wernicke's aphasia. *Brain and Language, 45,* 448–464.

SECTION II

2

A Case of Fluent Aphasia

Anna Basso and Audrey L. Holland

Case Description

MS, a 46-year-old Italian gentleman with a degree in statistics, experienced a stroke in April 2005. MS is an avid reader (books, newspapers, scientific papers), has a happy family (wife and two sons, 10 and 12 years old), and a rich social life. Being now unable to work he feels particularly unhappy because of his reading problems. MS was first seen in a rehabilitation service in May, 1 month postonset. His score on the Token test was 7/36 (cutoff score: 29/36; De Renzi & Faglioni, 1978); his speech was fluent with frequent phonological errors and rare verbal paraphasias. In a formal evaluation, his scores were all near zero (production of words and sentences, repetition of words, nonwords, and sentences, spontaneous writing and writing to dictation of words, nonwords, and sentences, reading aloud of words, nonwords, and sentences) except for word copying, and oral and written comprehension of words (80% correct) and short sentences (50% correct). He also had mild oral apraxia and scored 35/36 on the Raven's Colored Progressive Matrices (Raven, 1965).

Medical History

A CT-scan showed a large hypodense frontal-temporal-parietal area lesion extending to the basal ganglia in the left hemisphere. The neurologic examination performed a month later showed severe aphasia (detailed below), mild motor difficulty in using his right hand, and right hemisensory loss. No visual field deficits were observed.

Neuropsychological Evaluation

At 5 months postonset, MS was evaluated in the aphasia department in Milan, Italy. MS had a severe language disorder. His speech was fluent, prosody was good, and the rare sentences he produced spontaneously were grammatically correct; the most frequent errors were phonological, with word-finding difficulties and rare paraphasias.

The results of his neuropsychological evaluation (Table 2–1) showed that confrontation naming of actions and nouns were equal-

Table 1. WS: Aphasia Test Scores

Test	Score	Test	Score
Spoken Naming		*Repetition*	
Objects	20/60	Words	4/10
Actions	20/60	Nonwords	2/10
Written Naming			
Objects	42/60	*Writing to dictation*	
Actions	21/60	Words	4/10
Nonwords	2/10		
Auditory Verbal Comprehension		*Picture Description*	Phonemic and grammatical errors
Word-to-picture matching			
Oral	20/20		
Written	20/20	*Raven's Coloured Progressive Matrices*	53/60
Comprehension of short commands			
Oral	9/10		
Written	9/10	*Written calculation*	94/101
Comprehension of complex commands			
Token Test	13/36		

ly impaired (20% correct) with phonological errors (scala (stairs) →
salla), frequent false starts (bicchiere [glass] → bi bi ci-ci bi-ce-na;
fungo [mushroom] fa far fal fa falla), no responses, and nonwords
responses (campana [bell] → maponta). Errors were the same for
nouns and action verbs. Written confrontation naming was slight-
ly better than oral naming, and was better for nouns (70%) than actions (35%); errors were orthographic (orologio [watch] → orolo-
rio, ciliegia [cherry] → ciligra) for nouns; orthographic (mangiare
[to eat] → macire), no responses (scendere [to go down] → . . .),
and paraphasic (pettinare [to comb] → cappello [hat], tagliare [to
cut] → cucina [he cooks] for action verbs.

Oral and written word-picture matching of 20 words was 100%
correct, and oral and written comprehension of short commands
was 90% correct. Comprehension of more complex orders was severely impaired and he scored 13/36 on the Token Test.

He could repeat and write to dictation some words and nonwords but he scored 0% in sentence repetition and writing to dictation; errors were similar to those he makes in spontaneous speech
and writing. His reading was severely impaired and he could only
read a few simple words, when allowed time.

Description of a picture (sitting room with mother knitting,
father reading newspaper, girl watching TV, and boy playing with
wooden blocks) was as follows:

A A NON MI RICORDO; ANDAVA PER GIOCANDA; LA SIGNORA FA
FA MAIA (maglia); PICCOLA GUARDA LA LA TO TO TE TE GUARDA
QUA; QUESTO SIGNORE LEGGIA LEGGE; PICO PICCOLO FA GIO-
CA." (a a I don't remember; was going to playing [in Italian there is a
grammatical error (the preposition "per" requires the infinitive *gio-
care*], and a phonological error: it should have been "giocando"]; the
lady makes knitting [with a phonological error]; girl looks the the to
to te te [television] looks here; this man reads [with a phonological
error] reads [correct]; bo boy makes plays)

Written description of the same picture conveyed more or less
the same content but single graphemes errors were rarer than phonological errors and words were easily understandable ("gatto scoc-
cia! donna maglia! bambina televidore [television] uomo legge,
bambino cubo])" (cat annoys! woman stitch! girl television, man
reads, boy block").

He also had mild oral apraxia (no ideomotor apraxia); his score on the standard Raven's Progessive Matrices was very high (53/60), demonstrating largely unimpaired abstract thinking ability; his score on a written calculation task was in the normal range (94/101; cutoff score: 74/101).

References

De Renzi, E., & Faglioni, P. (1978). Normative data and screening power of a shortened version of the Token Test. *Cortex, 14,* 41–49.

Raven, J. C. (1965). *Guide to using the coloured matrices sets A, Ab, B.* London: H. K. Lewis.

Treatment for Fluent Aphasia from a Cognitive-Impairment Perspective

Anna Basso

Case Interpretation

The clinical diagnosis is not difficult: MS's speech is fluent with mainly phonological errors; comprehension and repetition are equally impaired. This description is consistent with Wernicke aphasia but it is possible to spot signs of "agrammatism" particularly in his written production: omission of function words and articles. Agrammatism is incompatible with a diagnosis of fluent aphasia but the existence of some variability among individuals classified as having the same syndrome is now acknowledged. Moreover, it must not be forgotten that only 20 to 30% of individuals with aphasia can be reliably classified in any of the classic aphasia syndromes (Albert, Goodglass, Helm, Rubens, & Alexander, 1981; Prins, Snow, & Wagenaar, 1978). This percentage is much higher if only vascular subjects in the subacute phase are considered. If, however, the concept of fluency is fundamental to reaching a correct clinical diagnosis, MS is unquestionably a Wernicke aphasic subject.

His aphasic disorder is severe but strikingly "pure"; except for very mild oral apraxia, no other cognitive impairment is present and his score on the standard Raven's progressive matrices, which are fairly demanding, is very high (52/60; Raven, 1938).

A clinical diagnosis is a useful tool for summarizing the subject's symptoms and for capturing some regularities of language disruption, but the clinical categories are too general to guide treatment. A theoretically justified and effective treatment must be based on a functional model of normal processing and be founded on a rational analysis of the subject's impairments. To locate MS's functional damage with reference to a model of normal language processing is, however, difficult because MS did not undergo a detailed and thorough examination. In a clinical setting it is not always possible to submit all subjects to a lengthy and demanding examination. Clinicians seldom have an opportunity to explore each subject's impairment systematically because of their heavy clinical caseloads.

Despite the limited data, an effort can be made to locate MS's impairments with reference to a model of the lexical-semantic system developed on the basis of studies of normal and brain-injured subjects and articulated as an information processing model. It presupposes the existence of a single semantic module and of four lexical components: the phonological input lexicon, the orthographic input lexicon, the phonological output lexicon, and the orthographic output. The input and output lexicons are connected with dedicated working memory systems (buffers); grapheme-to-phoneme and phoneme-to-grapheme conversion mechanisms allow reading and spelling of new words that, by definition, are not stored in the lexical components. A schematic representation of the structure of the lexical model that forms the basis for this discussion is depicted in Figure 3–1 and the characteristics of each component are briefly described below.

Graphemes and phonemes are abstract units and their physical realizations may have nothing in common. When hearing (or seeing) a word the incoming phonemes (or graphemes) must be identified and the string maintained in a working memory (buffer) in preparation for subsequent processing. The different realizations of a grapheme must be recognized as expressions of the same grapheme; "A, a, a" are physically different; they are recognized as different realizations of the grapheme [A] by the input graphemic buffer. Before addressing the lexicon, the buffer holds the graphemic string until it is completed. The phonological input buffer acts sim-

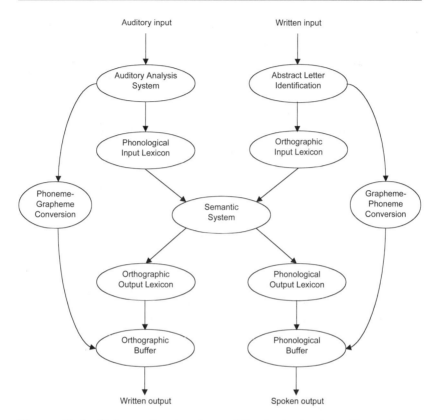

Figure 3–1. Schematic structure of the lexical-semantic system.

ilarly with the incoming phonemes and the input lexicon then processes the completed string.

The abstract phonological and orthographic representations of known words are stored in the input and output lexicons. The organization of the stored information is not completely understood but there are indications that words are organized by grammatical class and that root morphemes are separated from affixes. In the case of deficits in the lexicons, errors can show some lexical effects—such as a grammatical class effect—that can arise only at this level.

The semantic system contains stored knowledge about, among other phenomena, word meaning; it can be accessed from any input modality and can access any output modality. Semantic damage will cause problems performing any tasks that require semantic mediation and the errors will generally be semantic. The output buffers are short-term working memory systems that temporarily store representations in preparation for subsequent processes. The actual production of a word requires a given amount of time during which the abstract representation of the word must be continually reactivated for production to take place. Finally, normal literate subjects can read and spell novel words not stored in the lexicons; applying the conversion rules they can convert unforeseen sequences of graphemes into phonemes and vice versa.

The results of MS's language examination are now considered in reference to the model in order to locate the functional impairments.

Input Buffers

Processing of the input buffers, as of other lexical components, was not directly evaluated but the relatively spared repetition and spelling of nonwords and words and the unimpaired oral and written word-picture matching suggest good recognition of input phonemes and graphemes.

Input Lexicons

The task of choice for the evaluation of the input lexicons is lexical decision. A string of phonemes or graphemes is spoken or shown to the subject who has to decide whether or not the string corresponds to a known word. In the absence of direct evaluation, MS's 100% correct auditory and written word-picture matching can be taken as an indication of relatively well preserved input lexicons.

Semantic System

MS's semantic knowledge appears to be fairly preserved. In auditory and written word-picture matching tasks MS was 100% correct; in picture naming he made many phonological errors but the target word was generally recognizable and was the correct one in most cases. He produced two semantic paraphasias in action naming but his gestures showed that he knew that the response was not correct. Although this evidence is clearly not sufficient to rule out damage to the semantic system, it does preclude the possibility of finding severe damage.

Output Lexicons

The difference between better preserved word repetition (60%) and more severely damaged naming (25% for nouns and 20% for actions) cannot be explained by postlexical or semantic damage. Thus, the most plausible locus of damage is the phonological output lexicon. As for the orthographic output lexicon, the difference in writing nouns (70% correct) and action verbs (35% correct) points to damage at this level.

Output Buffers

MS made many phonological errors in all word and nonword production tasks, which can be taken as an indication of severe damage of the phonological output buffer. Similarly, damage to the graphemic output buffer can be inferred by the presence of orthographic errors in all words and nonwords spelling tasks.

Conversion Mechanisms

The data do not allow any conclusion about phoneme-to-grapheme conversion; difficulty in writing nonwords can be explained by damage to the output buffer only, but damage to the sublexical routine cannot be excluded. Grapheme-to-phoneme conversion mechanisms, on the other hand, seem to be impaired. MS's reading of nonwords was more severely impaired than his nonword repetition; this result cannot be explained by damage to the phonological output buffer only because the number of errors would be approximately the same in repetition and reading of nonwords. As the input buffer was grossly spared we must hypothesize damage to the conversion mechanisms.

In short, the input buffers, the input lexicons and the semantic system are grossly spared, the output lexicons and buffers are damaged, grapheme-to-phoneme conversion mechanisms are impaired, and no conclusion can be drawn about phoneme-to-grapheme conversion.

Data on sentence processing are limited and models of normal sentence processing are much less detailed than models of word processing, thus making it more difficult to locate the functional damage (but see Thompson, Chapter 11, this volume). As for comprehension, MS could only carry out some very simple commands, be they auditory or written, such as "blow your nose" or "open the book." He had a very low score on the Token Test, which has been shown to correlate well with severity of aphasia, but is not designed to locate the underlying functional damage, being based only on the idea that comprehension becomes more and more difficult with increasing information load.

If phonological errors are ignored, the following utterances are recognizable in his picture description: "I don't remember," "the lady makes knitting" (omission of an obligatory article in Italian), "girl watches TV" (omission of an obligatory article), "this man reads." Grammatical errors in writing are more evident; he omitted articles, prepositions, and verbs and used some verbs in the infinitive form.

To conclude, MS's sentence comprehension is severely impaired but it is not possible to hypothesize about the specific cause of the impairment. In speech production, MS apparently omitted articles; in writing he omitted articles, prepositions, and verbs.

Treatment

Output Buffers

The frequent and pervasive phonological errors are the most probable cause for the poor intelligibility of MS's speech; these errors are at least, in part, due to damage to the phonological buffer. Buffers are working memory components assigned to the temporary storage of lexical and nonlexical representations for successive elaboration. The nature of the stimulus—words or nonwords—should have no consequences but damage to a buffer will disclose a length effect and shorter stimuli will have a better chance of being correctly processed than longer ones. To treat the output buffer it seems sensible to use words as the output phonological lexicon was also damaged and needs treatment.

Both the phonological output lexicon and the phonological output buffer are accessed in reading aloud, repetition, and naming. MS's reading was the most impaired ability. Naming requires the subject to access the phonological form of the to-be-named word first, a difficult task for MS due to damage to the lexicon itself. Repetition, on the other hand, can be performed either via the input-to-output phoneme conversion route or the lexical route. It seems, therefore, well advised to ask MS to repeat words, concentrating all his efforts on the programming of the phonological plan. Initially, MS is to be required to repeat isolated words; short phrases can be added later when single words are correctly repeated. On hearing a word, he first has to pay attention to its meaning, sound out the word mentally, and focus upon its phonological form; when he is sufficiently sure he is correct, he is then to produce the word. If the response is not correct he should not try to correct it immediately but wait for a while, try to sound the word internally, and say it again. MS must be trained to program the phonological and articulatory plan of the to-be-produced word before saying it and to produce it only when reasonably sure to utter it correctly, in order to reduce as much as possible the number of errors.

After correct repetition, the word should be written. Writing words (and/or nonwords) under dictation is the exercise of choice for the rehabilitation of the output graphemic buffer and (in case of nonwords) of the phoneme-to-grapheme conversion rules. The main reason for asking MS to write the word is to train the graphemic output lexicon and buffer, but this activity also should maintain the subject's attention on the phonological form and spelling of the word and this should help to reinforce them—that is, their representation in memory. The length of the to-be-repeated word should be such as to have the subject make a consistent effort to repeat it correctly and it should be slowly increased as the subject progresses.

An important advantage of this exercise is that it can be easily carried out at home with the help of an untrained volunteer, such as the subject's spouse, a relative, or a friend.

Output Lexicons

One hopes the tasks described above would help MS make fewer phonological errors in speech and fewer errors in spelling words.

This, in turn, would permit those who work with him to better define the extent of damage to the output lexicons. The tasks, however, are not meant to tackle MS's word-finding-difficulties.

Naming disorders are a frequent and long-lasting deficit in aphasic subjects and various treatments have been described. Miceli, Amitrano, Capasso, and Caramazza (1996) presented the results of three different treatments for anomia in two chronic aphasic subjects; for both subjects damage was localized at the level of the phonological output lexicon. The three treatments consisted of repetition, reading aloud, and naming of a set of 30 words. All three methods gave positive results. The effect of repetition, reading aloud, and an orthographic cue in learning words was compared in normal subjects and two aphasic individuals by Basso, Marangolo, Piras, and Galluzzi (2001). The orthographic cue was shown to be the most effective learning method, confirming the generation effect (Slamecka & Graft, 1978): the more effortful technique is more effective than the less effortful methods. It seems fair to conclude that training on any task that requires the oral production of the to-be-treated words should result in improvement in subjects with damage to the phonological output lexicon and spared semantics, but that some methods are more effective than others.

Therefore, I would ask MS to write down, with the aid of the therapist, the name of a depicted object (his written naming was better than his oral naming); when the written word is completed he should produce it orally, always sounding it internally before saying it, so as not to make phonological errors. The aim of this exercise is to improve the phonological lexicon, but writing of the word necessarily involves the orthographic output lexicon and buffer. Partial recovery of these components, even if not directly tackled, may also be improved.

Naming to confrontation, although efficacious, is suggested only for severely anomic subjects. When anomia is moderate, naming to confrontation is not the task of choice because only a limited number of words are picturable, because anomia is a persistent disorder that requires intensive and protracted therapy, and finally because preserved confrontation naming does not guarantee that the subject will use the words he or she can name to confrontation in spontaneous speech.

Confrontation naming tasks should be abandoned as soon as possible and MS should work at home with a small dictionary with a reduced number of words and easy definitions. Starting with any letter he chooses to start with, every day MS should underline three to four words (starting with nouns, verbs and adjectives) that he thinks useful for him at the moment, read the words aloud, read the definitions (MS had a severe deficit in reading aloud but his comprehension of written words is relatively well preserved and it would be sufficient for him to pick up some words), repeat the word silently, write it down, and then say it. MS should spend 2 to 3 hours per day on this task that has been shown to be efficacious when carried out for many months (Basso, 2005).

If these exercises are successful, MS's speech will contain fewer phonological errors and his naming will improve. At the same time, the orthographic output lexicon and the orthographic output buffer, not directly dealt with but included in all tasks, should partially recover.

Improvement of the orthographic output lexicon is expected also on the basis of results of a different treatment that was shown to be effective in normal subjects (Basso, Burgio, & Prandoni, 1999) and in an aphasic individual (Berhmann & Herdan, 1987). Basso et al. (1999) asked 20 normal controls without previous knowledge of French to learn spellings of 12 French words that could not be written by Italian correspondence rules. The examiner said the word while the subjects looked at the written word. When asked to write them for the first time, the subjects learning of a consistent number of words. The authors advanced the hypothesis that this was done by conjuring up the written representation of the word in a visual buffer and copying the word from the buffer. A similar method was used in the rehabilitation of CCM (Berhmann & Herdan, 1987), a surface dysgraphic, who was asked to select the correct form of a written word from several alternatives. MS is asked to look up a word in the dictionary, read the definition, and write down the word. This obviously keeps the subject's attention on the written form of the word and may help recovery of the orthographic output lexicon.

Grapheme-to-Phoneme Conversion

Reading of words and nonwords is the most severely impaired ability. Damage to the phonological output lexicon and the phonological output buffer is sufficient to explain impaired reading of words and treatment of these components has already been described. Impaired reading of nonwords is partially explained by damage to the phonological output buffer but damage to the conversion mechanisms has also been hypothesised. I would, however, postpone treatment of grapheme-to-phoneme conversion mechanisms, notwithstanding the fact that MS is an avid reader and complains of not being able to read. This is because of the massive effort required to address impairments of the output lexicons and buffers that are the most devastating for his communication capacity. Only later should nonword reading be taken into consideration. This can be done by asking the subject to read simple CV syllables in which the vowel is held constant; when this task is mastered it can be made more difficult by presenting short nonwords made up by 3 graphemes or 2 CVCV syllables. Italian has a transparent orthography and almost every word can be read by conversion rules. This renders recovery of grapheme-to-phoneme conversion easier than in other languages that do not have a transparent orthography, like English. The task can be done at home with the help of a relative and this allows for intensive practice.

Sentences

As lexical disorders clear, there should be a better understanding of MS's sentence disorders that should then be taken into account. It is difficult to suggest any treatment for MS's sentence disorders now since, as stated earlier, no thorough analysis is possible, mainly because of the severity of his lexical impairments.

Outcome

We know from the literature that improvement of the orthographic output lexicon, the phonological output lexicon, the phonological output buffer, the orthographic output buffer, and grapheme-to-phoneme conversion rules is possible, and some examples of successful treatments are given below. Treatments have been described that appear to be effective for reactivating or rebuilding orthographic output representations (Beeson, 1999; Beeson, Hirsch,

& Rewega, 2002; Rapp & Kane, 2002). Rapp and Kane (2002), for instance, successfully used a delayed copying technique; their subjects looked at the written word while the clinician read the letter, and then had to write the word. We have already seen that different techniques—reading aloud, repetition, orthographic cue—may be successful in the rehabilitation of the phonological output lexicon (Basso et al., 1999; Miceli et al., 1996).

Improvement of the orthographic output lexicon and the phonological output lexicon tends to be restricted to trained words without generalization to untrained words. This is consistent with the idea of the lexicon as a store; the abstract phonological and orthographic representations of known words must be restored one by one. Lack of generalization is the main reason why it is suggested to use a dictionary and work intensively for months or even years, at least for as long as it is possible to show acquisition of new words.

As for treatment of an impaired phonological output buffer, Pradat-Diehl et al. (2001) successfully treated an aphasic subject with conduction aphasia and impaired phonological output buffer. The treatment was intensive (5 and then 3 sessions per week with the clinician and 4 hours per day at home). The subject was asked to imagine the written word he wanted to say, "read" it very slowly, and produce it one syllable at a time. A semantic technique was also employed: before saying the last word of a sentence, the subject was asked to say whether or not the sentence made sense, thus giving him time to think and internally process the word.

Cardell and Chenery (1999) asked their subject with an output graphemic buffer impairment to write four-letter nonwords under dictation. The subject received treatment twice weekly; treatment was discontinued when he correctly wrote 80% of the treated items. Improvement of the treated items began after 5 sessions and generalization to untreated items occurred, confirming that therapy had targeted the impaired process rather than individual items.

Treatment of the grapheme-to-phoneme conversion rules has frequently been carried out in subjects with deep dyslexia (e.g., De Partz, 1986). Greenwald (2004) trained grapheme-to-phoneme conversions in a subject—MM—with severe global agraphia. A first set of 7 graphemes was trained and then a second set and training continued until MM reached 100% accuracy. MM learned the first set of 7 graphemes in 9 sessions and the second set in 6 sessions.

It is expected that MS will show good recovery because he is highly motivated, ready to work hard on his problems, and suffers from a "pure" aphasia unaccompanied by other cognitive disorders (with the possible exception of mild oral apraxia), unless, of course, the proposed exercises are completely mistaken. Moreover, MS is required to work intensively with the aid of his spouse, a relative, or a friend for treatment of the phonological output buffer damage, and on his own with a small dictionary to overcome his output lexicon deficits. This is important because it has been repeatedly shown that intensity and duration of treatment are important factors for recovery (e.g., Basso, 2005).

Finally, whenever possible errors are avoided and there are hints that errorless learning is more efficacious than trial and error learning (Wilson, Baddeley, Evans, & Shiel, 1994). If MS's lexical disorders improve, a better evaluation of his sentence processing disorders will be easier and will probably allow a rational intervention to be implemented. It is also expected that improvement of the impaired components will immediately show up in MS's communication capacity in his daily life. MS's behavior in conversation was normal; he understood the fact that in a conversation people have different roles – listener and speaker – that change continuously; he was clearly interested in conversation exchanges and was able to understand (as long as his interlocutor did not use rare words or difficult grammatical constructions) what the topic of the conversation was. His communication capacity was hampered by his lexical (and probably syntactic) deficits but his pragmatic competence was normal, as would be the pragmatic competence of a normal subject trying to communicate in a little known language.

Summary

In suggesting therapy for MS, an effort has been made to relate the tasks to the underlying deficits. In the history of aphasia therapy, reference to an explicit model of normal processing has not always formed the basis of the treatments. Skilled and intuitive clinicians have devised successful methods that have become part of each clinician equipment. Lack of a clear relationship between the impairment and the treatment, however, prevents understanding why the treatment has been efficacious and to extend the same treatment to other subjects who will never be exactly the same as the first, successfully treated, subject. Our practical experience will be enriched but our theoretical knowledge will not be furthered.

The standard approach to treatment poses serious problems in the evaluation of the efficacy of aphasia therapy because no principled reasons to favor the intervention methods employed can be found. I am not arguing that tasks different from the ones proposed here would not be equally or even more efficacious but I am claiming that in order to develop and support hypotheses about why a treatment is effective, therapy should be logically linked to the theoretical interpretation of the impairment and should constrain the selection of the therapeutic procedures.

References

Albert, M. L., Goodglass, H., Helms, N. A., Rubens, A. B., & Alexander, M. P. (1981). *Clinical aspects of dysphasia.* Wien: Springer-Verlag.

Basso, A. (2005). How intensive/prolonged should an intensive/prolonged treatment be? *Aphasiology, 19,* 975–984.

Basso, A., Burgio, F., & Prandoni P. (1999). Acquisition of output irregular orthographic representations in normal adults: An experimental study. *Journal of the International Neuropsychological Society, 5,* 405–412.

Basso, A., Marangolo, P., Piras, F., & Galluzzi, C. (2001). Acquisition of new words in normal subjects: A suggestion for the treatment of anomia. *Brain and Language, 77,* 45–59.

Beeson, P. M. (1999). Treating acquired writing impairment: Strengthening graphemic representations. *Aphasiology, 13,* 367–386.

Beeson, P. M., Hirsch, F., & Rewega, M. (2002). Successful single words writing treatment: Experimental analysis of four cases. *Aphasiology, 16,* 473–491.

Behrmann, M., & Herdan, S. (1987). The case for cognitive neuropsychological rehabilitation. *Die Suid-Afrikaanse Tydschift vir Kommunikasieafwykings, 34,* 3–9.

Cardell, E.A., & Chenery, H.J. (1999). A cognitive neuropsychological approach to the assessment and remediation of acquired dysgraphia. *Language Testing, 16,* 353–388.

De Partz, M-P. (1986). re-education of a deep dyslexic patient: rationale of the method and results. *Cognitive Neuropsychology, 3,* 149–177.

Greenwald, M. (2004). "Blocking" lexical competitors in severe global agraphia: A treatment of reading and spelling. *Neurocase, 10,* 156–174.

Miceli, G., Amitrano, A., Capasso, R., & Caramazza, A. (1996). The treatment of anomia from output lexical damage: Analysis of two cases. *Brain and Language, 52,* 150-174.

Pradat-Diehl, P., Tessier, C., Vallat, C., Mailhan, L., Mazevet, D., Lauriot-Prevost, M.C., Bergego, C. (2001). Aphasie de conduction par trouble phonémique. *Revue Neurologique, 157,* 1245-1252.

Prins, R. S., Snow, C. E., & Wagenaar E. (1978). Recovery from aphasia: Spontaneous speech versus language comprehension. *Brain and Language, 5,* 192-211.

Rapp, B., Kane, A. (2002). Remediation of deficits affecting different components of the spelling process. *Aphasiology, 16,* 439-454.

Raven, J. C. (1938). *Standard progressive matrices: Sets A, B, C, D & E.* London: H. K. Lewis.

Slamecka, N. J., Graf, P. (1978). The generation effect: Delineation of a phenomenon. *Journal of Experimental Psychology: Human Learning and Memory, 4,* 592-604.

Wilson, B., Baddeley, A., Evans, J., & Shiel, A. (1994). Errorless learning in the rehabilitation of memory impaired people. *Neuropsychological Rehabilitation, 4,* 307-326.

Concentrating on the Consequences

Consequence-Oriented Treatment

Audrey L. Holland

Introduction

In Chapter 3, Dr. Basso provided information concerning the nature of the cerebral event, the language testing data and some demographic details concerning MS, who is the focal point of our varying treatments. Dr. Basso has also permitted me to add to MS's psychosocial profile some details that are apocryphal, but necessary for some of the fine points of the treatment approach I will outline below.

I have had the pleasure of reading Dr. Basso's treatment plan, which is thorough and well grounded in prevailing theories of neurocognitive functioning. In this chapter, I do not draw the reader into argument, but simply present a different focus. Following in Dr. Basso's footsteps, I describe the way I would approach MS's treatment, giving its rationale and presenting illustrative exercises when appropriate along the way. I have assumed that I am the treating clinician. It is one thing to prescribe what others are supposed to do; it is invariably less grandiose when I assume that I am the one who must follow through.

Additional Information for Consequences-Oriented Treatment

All of Dr. Basso's information is necessary. It provides a universally understood description of MS's aphasia. However, for a clinician whose therapeutic focus is on the consequences of this aphasia on his everyday life, more information is required.

This additional information relates to understanding not only MS's aphasia, but also MS as a person. Shadden has described aphasia as "identity theft" (2005); one of my treatment goals concerns helping MS and his family to re-assert their senses of self. Thus, before I begin to work with MS, I need to know more about him, his passions, his more minor enthusiasms, his opinions, his dislikes, and some clues about his resilience. It is also useful to know about his family and the nature of family relationships. Because he is relatively young, with a young family, and probably nearing the peak of his career (and earning power), there is a particular urgency and costliness about what must be a catastrophic family loss. In my view, understanding the family dynamic as well as the person with aphasia is critical to good management and, in fact, may be more important than understanding the nature of the language loss itself.

Therefore, I have included additional psychosocially relevant information concerning MS. MS was employed as an officer of a major bank in Milan. He is moderately depressed since the stroke, but his history suggests that he and Mrs. MS have a strong, supportive relationship. He is a serious reader, whose interests include opera, current events, and mysteries. He is an avid soccer fan. MS, his wife, and two sons are devoted skiers who traditionally spend the Christmas holidays at a ski resort. MS' degree in statistics foreshadows his mathematical abilities and interests, which appear to be relatively intact.

Mrs. MS is a lawyer, who works full time in city government. It will be possible for her to adjust her responsibilities to permit her to participate in his treatment. Both Mr. and Mrs. MS come from large families who live nearby, and their families are available to help in his rehabilitation. (The family is largely supportive and involved. If the family were less supportive, less able to be of help, and so on, the therapy that follows would reflect those additional concerns.)

To be consistent with the time frame of treatment proposed by Dr. Basso, MS comes to my clinic for treatment for his aphasia 5 months poststroke. Thus his therapy during more acute stages will not be emphasized here. (Incidentally, this is not an uncommon time for individuals with aphasia to begin therapy of the type to be discussed here. They have often finished their inpatient rehabilitation, which has probably focused more explicitly on the language impairment, typically run out of benefits, in the United States at least, and although even substantial improvement may have occurred, face residual difficulties in communication.)

Underlying Assumptions

The proposed therapy assumes three things:

1. "Expertise" as it applies to aphasia treatment is shared by the aphasic person, the family, and the clinician. All must be included in therapy planning and focus.
2. Therapy builds on strengths, as opposed to limitations, with the goal of buttressing strengths.
3. To the extent possible, therapy incorporates interests. Each is discussed below.

The Concept of Shared Expertise

In relation to the treatment of aphasia, this concept has been well explored by a number of writers including Parr and Byng (2000) and Worrall (1999, 2000). Shared expertise is a logical extension of some concerns of the Disability Movement regarding the active involvement of disabled people and their close ones in care and management. Its implications for aphasia treatment concern mutual, informed, decision-making by the relevant experts: the person with aphasia who is living *in* the problem; the family, who is living *with* the problem; and the clinician, who brings broad experience and knowledge *to*the problem. Ideally, all should share in making decisions concerning where therapy should be heading, what are reasonable goals, what constitute the most nagging and thorniest of problems, and so on. Their varying influence probably differs at differing time points in recovery, with clinician expertise dominating early when family and aphasic individuals are bewildered, possibly panicked, and when they may never have heard the word "aphasia." In such circumstances, a cardinal responsibility of the clinician is to provide support and information about the disorder. Similarly, early rehabilitation might well be focused on lessening the impairment of aphasia, and helping the family to cope. The balance of expertise gradually shifts as time goes on; as patients and families live into the disorder, they begin to assert their expertise. Timing may not be everything, but it is certainly important, and by 5 months poststroke, MS and his family are beginning to realize that, although his language abilities have improved to a substantial degree, and they will likely continue on that course for a while, aphasia is likely to be a chronic problem. Some energy must now be directed toward learning to live successfully with the disorder. The fact of lingering, significant aphasia is also likely to be an important player in MS's depression. Thus, involving the family in treatment planning seems mandatory. What do all three bring to the management of MS's aphasia?

MS brings his lifelong interests, and his elemental understanding of what aphasia is costing him in terms of his lifestyle and life goals. He also brings his own motivation, a factor that I do not believe others are well placed to estimate. Family members are often surprised by an aphasic individual's drive and tenacity, or by a willingness to accept the consequences of stroke. (Incidentally, "acknowledgement" or "fitting aphasia in" are, to my way of thinking, important factors in learning to move on.) I am assuming here that, despite depression, MS is interested in getting on with his life, particularly in relation to preserving his parental role with his sons. He also seems very motivated to improve his reading. Whether he can resume his career as a bank officer is entirely unclear, and now is not the time for making such a decision.

The family appears to bring an understanding of their own family dynamics, and the fact that this appears to be a well-functioning family is a strong positive factor. Nevertheless, family issues, including the effects of aphasia on two relatively young children, MS's possible feelings of inadequacy in helping them to grow up, and potential lifestyle changes brought about by the possibility of early retirement and reduced income, role reversals, and so on, all influence the course and direction of treatment. The wise clinician recognizes that MS is only one of a family constellation affected by his aphasia. Its effects on family and children are at least as important.

What does the third expert, the clinician, contribute? First and very importantly, a broad understanding and knowledge of aphasia and its treatment. For example, I know a variety of approaches to treatment that might be useful here. I have relatively firm understanding of theories of language processing that provide useful approaches to the treatment of aphasia. Finally, I know that all of the above information is likely to influence and affect treatment, and that I need to remain sensitive to it.

So what do our three experts believe are important intervention goals? MS's immediate goals are to (1) improve his ability to understand speech and to regain confidence in his ability to comprehend the world around him; (2) be able to read again at a level that will permit him to read newspapers and some fiction; and (3) participate more actively in family life. Mrs. MS's goals for her husband are compatible with his, but her personal goal is to become comfortable in leaving him alone while she works. I agree with these goals, but with the stipulation that he and the family agree to devote a substantial amount of time and effort to reaching them. I am explicit about making no guarantees.

Building on Strengths.

Both communicative strengths and personal strengths count. In MS's case, it is easy to identify his personal strengths. Specifically, they include his age, and his intelligence. Despite his depression, he appears to be well motivated especially regarding re-establishing reading. MS seems to respond well to challenge, and is both affable and gregarious.

Regarding language, I would concentrate on his reading, because it is his major interest, but primarily because MS'a single-word reading is good, and I have grown up in a tradition, going back to Eisenson and Schuell, that stresses the importance of capitalizing on reading when comprehension of spoken speech is compromised. Reading, in effect, becomes a route to "getting through." It has an additional advantage of facilitating auditory comprehension to some degree. Because single-word speaking, and writing are also within MS's capabilities, they can serve as a secondary treatment focus. Finally, because of his mathematical background and his apparently intact number skills, I would take advantage of them in planning activities for treatment. Treatment will not explicitly include tasks aimed at improving auditory comprehension, per se. Rather, ensuring adequate comprehension will be an accompaniment of *every* treatment activity.

Incorporating Interests

Incorporating the interests of aphasic individuals in treatment is sometimes challenging. However, in addition to the importance of personal relevance in ensuring the aphasic person's involvement in the treatment process, it also helps to maintain clinician involvement. Taking clients' interests into account provides the clinician with sources of new information and new pleasures. I have learned a lot from my clients. The new things they have taught me have helped me to avoid burnout. MS's interests have already been noted, and they are featured in this approach to his treatment.

Therapy Plan

Influenced by a growing literature (Bhogul, Teasel, & Foley, 2003; Hinckley & Craig, 1998; Raymer et al., in press), I am convinced that intensity of treatment is a serious factor that influences outcome positively. I have the good fortune here to be writing about an Italian individual, for whom intensive treatment might be easier to obtain than were MS an American person. Thus, the regimen will include 5 days of treatment weekly. It will be a collaborative effort involving MS and his family, and will include group participation, one-on one intervention, lots of homework, and family involvement. Each is described briefly below.

Groups

Ideally, MS would be involved in 3 or 4 days of group treatment, consuming 3 or more hours each day. I have in mind centers for aphasia support such as those provided by the California Aphasia Center, the Aphasia Institute, the Adler Center, or UK Connect. (Web sites for these venters are included in the Appendix 4A.) Absent such programs, less intense group experiences, grounded in concern for psychosocial issues, may serve as reasonable, if paler, substitutes. Spouse group attendance by Mrs. MS would also be helpful, and hopefully such support groups are available as well.

There are a number of reasons why group treatment seems appropriate for both MS and his spouse. His aphasia has begun to assume a chronic, if still malleable, form. Thus they are beginning to face the psychosocial issues that surround living successfully with chronic aphasia. Groups are particularly useful in this regard, especially when one takes MS's reactive depression into account. Groups are beneficial environments for learning that one is not alone, that others have been in similar places, and can be of help as one finds one's own way.

There are many relevant examples of this group power. Here are two comments from aphasic individuals about this issue. My client RR noted that he felt he really did not begin to get better until he had begun group participation (Holland, 2007). He remained involved in groups for the rest of his life. Another aphasic individual described what he gained from his experiences in aphasia groups as a "psychic boost" (Moore, 1994).

There are other advantages to groups as well. Conversation opportunities are standard in groups, and will permit MS to try out his emerging skills in a supportive, natural environment. Thus, groups are a step toward normalization of social interaction. There is also evidence that groups themselves can foster decreases in aphasia severity (Elman & Bernstein-Ellis, 1999). Finally Mrs. MS's participation in spouse/partner groups is presumed to have similar advantages, at least the psychosocial ones, although the research on this topic is surprisingly scanty.

To gain a full picture of group treatment, and its scope, readers are urged to consult Elman (2007). This book presents an in-depth account of the diversity of group experiences available for adults and families with neurogenic communication disorders.

One-on-One Intervention

As noted earlier, MS does relatively well at the single-word level in terms of speaking, reading, and writing. I would choose to focus primarily on reading single words early on. Silent reading is the first target, then reading aloud, which will bring speech into the process.

Although it will be seen later that an innovative procedure will be incorporated, many of these activities are relatively mundane. The difference is that they focus on words and concepts that have resonance in MS's daily life. This is a relatively primitive notion, but one that is frequently overlooked particularly in individual therapy. If it is true that one learns what one practices, (virtually no data refute this), then, for tasks such as these, single words that one actually might want, and have occasion, to use seem a logical focus.

Traditional Practice

I would focus on reading single words relevant to family (family names are foremost), followed by personally salient words such as favorite restaurants and other activities that have some likelihood of being currently pertinent. For example, words related to the Torino Olympics, skiing terms and destinations, names of soccer teams, players, scores, operas, singers, conductors, and so forth. Following is an example, from La Scala:

Stimulus materials could be a set of 3×5 cards, with names of opera events, participants, and so forth.

▓ Example tasks: Separate male and female principal singers. Once done, correctly (feedback given) then they should be read silently, then read aloud.Separate operas on the most recent schedule from those that are not. Read silently, then read aloud, and so forth. Separate into favorite versus other opera titles, singers, and so on, using the same protocol

Once single-word reading on a variety of tasks such as these is mastered, new and additional index cards would follow. Cards are now used to fill in slots in simple sentences, with three or four alternatives.

▓ For example, _____ _____ was booed from the stage during last Sunday's performance of Aïda.

Tasks can proceed with increasing complexity. It is important to note that recent experimental work in aphasia (Kiran & Thompson, 2003; Thompson 2007; Thompson, Shapiro, Kiran, & Sobeks, 2003) has shown that there is value in working at an appropriately high level of complexity to permit generalization to easier tasks. (See Chapter 7 for a relevant example.) This is one reason why I am not bothered by the low frequency of the words we are working with, above. Initially, accuracy is more important than speed, but once accuracy is achieved, then it is permissible to work toward more timely responding. When stimuli are both semantically challenging and personally relevant, as accuracy is achieved, it is also possible to progress in complexity. The goal of such work, of course, is to facilitate reading newspapers and books.

Reading tasks incorporating math skills would also be used. These might include making change, and price tag reading, progressing to balancing accounts with the goal of re-establishing one of MS's previous household roles.

Conversation

A substantial part of each treatment hour must be devoted to conversation. Goals for these daily conversations are varied. Conversation provides an opportunity for the clinician to check frequently on the generalization of MS's formal treatment to the most important arena—that of becoming a communication partner again. Conversation also provides the best opportunity to observe and to reinforce the strategies and techniques MS uses to help him to get his message across to others when verbal communication alone is unsatisfactory, or to teach him how to generalize the use of effective strategies to real world interaction. Finally, conversation humanizes the therapy process and provides an opportunity for communication counseling (see Holland, 2007). If the clinician devalues conversation by failing to participate in it with the client, she sends a bewildering and mixed message to her client, at best.

Innovative and Experimental Approaches

As knowledge of effective treatments grows, it is important for clinicians to be alert for those that can potentially have an impact on a particular client.[1] In the case of MS, at least two seem applicable;

---

[1]A side benefit of suggesting and incorporating innovative approaches is that, for many aphasic individuals, it provides the satisfaction of being involved in treatment that is "on the cutting-edge." This is often an intrinsic motivator, particularly evident when innovative treatments are undertaken as part of a clinical trial, or when information concerning an individual's progress with the approach are, with agreement, made available to the pertinent researcher.

I would investigate both or, at some point in his therapy regimen, incorporate trial sessions of each. These two approaches are Constraint-Induced Language Therapy (CILT) (Maher, Kendall, Swearengen, et al., in press; Pulvermueller, Neininger, Elbert, et al, 2001) and the preparation and use of scripts for training short relevant monologues, or participation in dialogues (Youmans, Holland, Munoz, & Bourgeois, 2005). Each is described briefly below.

CILT, as described by Maher et al., (in press) incorporates a PACE-like format (i.e., Promoting Aphasics Communicative Effectiveness) (Davis and Wilcox, 1985), with new information sent in barrier-game tasks. Two aphasic individuals serve as partners in sending and receiving information. CILT differs from typical PACE in that the information to be shared across the barrier must be verbal. The clinician using CILT acts to facilitate the message sender, buttressing his or her verbal attempts, and if need be, even whispering the verbal message to be sent in order that the client may repeat it. Data are currently emerging to support gains in spoken language following CILT training.

Scripting was originally conceived as a way to enhance fluent output in individuals with nonfluent aphasia. The aphasic speaker and the clinician jointly prepare personally relevant scripts on topics of the speaker's choice. These scripts might be monologues such as a favorite family story, a short speech, or directions to one's house. Dialogue scripts can be formulaic exchanges of greetings and questions to use in conversations, say with one's grandchildren, over the telephone; they might also be one's answers to a highly ritualized dialogue such as ordering a pizza over the phone. Guidelines for how to prepare scripts can be found in Youmans et al. (2005.) or in Holland and Ramage (2004). Once generated, scripts are prepared in audiotape or written form, and sent home for intensive practice. Typically an agreement is forged as to the amount of time that will be devoted to script practice, and a log of actual use is kept. Work at the Rehabilitation Institute of Chicago to automate the script preparation and presentation is currently underway (Cherney, Halper, Holland, & Cole, in press). This automated version appears to be useful with fluent aphasias, in addition to the nonfluent speakers for whom it was initially designed.

Homework

I earlier noted a growing consensus about the increased effectiveness of intensive language/communication intervention. Because intensive experiences such as those available at aphasia centers are rare, other ways to achieve intensity (and systematicity) of treatment should be sought. Both the innovative approaches described above have been designed for intensive intervention.

Whether or not innovative approaches are incorporated into treatment, a regimen of consistent, daily homework should be undertaken. I am not advocating the use of generic practice workbooks that are frequently translated by clinicians into "homework." These workbooks lack the qualities of personal relevance that engage interest and attention, and often appear to be relatively abstract, even boring, drills.

Homework activities that are relevant for consequences-oriented aphasia treatment should be interesting, personally appropriate, and present opportunities of individuals to note their own progress. One of the most important is keeping a daily journal, and I would require MS to do so. As time goes on, the journal will become a record of progress, obvious to the aphasic individual and his or her family. For MS, early journal entries might consist simply of copying family member names, but grow over time to include, first, self-generated words, then to short comments on his day, and so forth. Incidentally, I never correct journals. I might comment on them, or suggest that the writer think about correcting his or her own. But they remain personal journals.

Television, newspapers (large print, if necessary) and, above all, the Internet, can provide effective homework tasks. For example, I might assign MS to watch two soccer games each week, and enter into his journal some important details about the game (opposing team, who won, who scored goals, league standing, and so forth. He should be encouraged to use the Web sites of local teams to help him search for details, not only for use in his homework, but to take advantage of the Internet's vast resources for augmenting his therapy. I also might ask him to look up a few words each day on an Internet dictionary, and to enter them into his journal. I would encourage the use of e-mail as soon as formulaic messages (perhaps taught before scripting techniques) can be entered, and whenever MS can access it comfortably. MS has already begun to use the Internet, but as progress is made, task difficulty should be increased; for example, after watching soccer on TV, he might use Internet reports of the game to write brief, previously formatted reports.

Newspaper activities might include finding and tracking and recording the performances of some of his favorite stocks (e.g., Prada, Menarini, and Fiat) on the stock market, or checking the La Scala schedule to record the names of at least two operas and two of its principal singers onstage each week.

As treatment progresses, homework should progress, too. For example, MS likes to read mysteries, and his favorite writer turns out to be Carlo Lucarelli. Once some reading ability is re-established, I would start with a Lucarelli mystery he has already read and liked, and have him read it aloud in accompaniment with that book on tape. Then he could move on to previously unread ones, with audiotape support, and over time, the audiotape is removed

Those who are involved in MS's recovery, of course, must support such activities by asking about them, sharing them, using them as the bases for conversation, and remarking on change and progress. The assignments are not casual; rather, they are to be considered part of the fabric of MS's treatment. They also make a logical transition point for the last topic of this chapter, family involvement.

Families and Rehabilitation

An implicit feature of consequences-oriented treatment is that the family is an important part of the rehabilitation process. But the family is also directly affected by aphasia, sometimes needing attention in its own right. Both aspects of family work will be discussed briefly.

Involving the Family

The "quickest fix" available in aphasia rehabilitation is to train the family to enhance the communication of their aphasic family member. In a nutshell, when individuals who interact with aphasic persons know how to buttress and enhance the aphasic person's communicative efforts, the likelihood of communicative success is increased. In fact, aphasic people communicate more effectively when trained partners scaffold their efforts. Perhaps the most widely known and practiced approach is to teach principles of Supported Communication, as described by Kagan and colleagues (Kagan, 1999; Kagan & Gailey, 1993). Deceptively clear-cut and simple, most of the supporting techniques that are involved, such as, providing appropriate time, providing useful cues, reminding individuals of what might enhance their communicative efforts, and so forth, require observation and practice by communication partners. Clinicians must provide practice time, demonstrate the effects of supported communication, and systematically teach families to use appropriate supports. In most cases, lists of do's and don'ts, although useful, are a poor substitute for demonstration and practice.

One way to provide practice is to formalize the use of appropriate communicative strategies by both the individual who has aphasia and his relevant family members. One such approach, "conversational coaching" (Hopper, Holland, & Rewega 2003) was developed in our laboratory over a number of years. Essentially coaching involves a clinician providing fresh information—a personal story, a video clip, a reprise of some event—to an aphasic person. The clinician then helps him to communicate its content by determining and then practicing appropriate strategies. Once the message is practiced, the aphasic person shares the message with a listener (family member) who is unfamiliar with the content. The clinician now acts as a coach for both the aphasic person and the family member, suggesting ways for each to provide more detailed cues, encouragers, and so forth. This procedure is practiced, with different messages and stories, until both participants are comfortable with it and demonstrate increased communicative effectiveness.

Conversational coaching seems particularly appropriate for MS, as it would be possible to involve not only his spouse, but also other family members, particularly his children, in learning and applying these techniques. Sessions typically are light in tone, and the processes are easily grasped. Regardless of the approach chosen, teaching family members to enhance communication is an important ingredient in consequence-focused treatment.

Beeke, Maxim, and Wilkinson (2007) have recently developed an observational procedure, analyzed by conversational analysis, whereby they train aphasic individuals and their spouses to converse more effectively. The procedure is straightforward, and seems easy to implement. I would certainly consider this approach in the management of conversation between MS and his spouse.

Supporting the Family

Avent, Glista, Wallace, et al. (2005) studied family-member focus groups who reported their concerns about aphasia at onset, during rehabilitation and following discharge from formal rehabilitation. Clinicians can use these focus group reports to structure their family interventions. Table 4-1 provides a list of the focus group concerns that were related to chronic aphasia, that is after discharge from formal rehabilitation. Such questions are likely to be the concerns of families such as that of MS.

Note that these questions approach practical problems in living with disability, not entirely focused on aphasia, but on how to get along despite it. The wise clinician should be prepared to help the family to get answers to them.

One particular issue that warrants attention in the MS family is the presence of two fairly young children, and the effects of aphasia on them and on MS's ability to fulfill his established parenting role. There is no indication that this is a particular problem, but the clinician should be alert to that potential. In that regard, please remember that the MS family took skiing vacations before aphasia entered their lives. Because MS has only minimal physical disabilities since his stroke, exploring the notion of resuming this tradition, and perhaps encouraging the planning of such a trip might be an appropriate source of stimulus material for direct therapy.

As suggested earlier, I am a strong believer in family support groups. They sometimes provide opportunities for families simply

Table 4–1. Concerns of a Focus Group of Spouses of Individuals with Chronic Aphasia.

What alterative therapies or activities are available?

Who can we call when we have questions?

What else can help at home?

Where can we get travel information?

Is job training available?

What support services are available?

What resources are available for long-range planning?

Source: From "Family information needs about aphasia," by J. Avent, S. Glista, S. Wllace, J. Jackson, J. Nisioka, and W. Yip in *Aphasiology, 19,* 365-375. Copyright 2005 Aphasiology. Reprinted with permission.

to get away from aphasia temporarily, but they also provide an opportunity to focus on family problems post aphasia, to learn from others, and to find common ground with others through sharing experiences and stories. A group of family members bring mutual expertise and problem solving that typically outweighs that of the clinician in charge.

However, if face-to-face support groups are not available, there is a plethora of principled material available on the Internet (in English at least) where families can find support. A selection of relevant Web sites are included in Appendix 4A.. Most of these Web sites have links to resource materials designed for families and individuals poststroke and living with aphasia. One particularly important example is the *Aphasia Handbook,* originally published for use in the United Kingdom by UK Connect (see Web site in Appendix 4A), but recently modified for use in the United States (Sarno & Peters, 2004). It is singled out here because it contains such extensive usable information for families and individuals living with aphasia. In addition, the fact that it has undergone a successful cultural translation might inspire individuals living in other countries to make similar translations. Finally, there are a number of works, written by aphasic people, or about aphasic people that provide support and help. One particularly useful example of this type is Eileen Quann's story of her husband's aphasia (2002).

Summary

I have tried to provide a template for how I might approach and conduct aphasia treatment focused on its consequences. It is certainly far from *rocket* science. However, it is not far from *linguistic* science and I have attempted to create an interplay between a language impairment itself, and language in interaction.

I am concerned with how aphasic persons manage their language problems, but also with how they manage to live with aphasia. Aphasia seldom goes away, despite our best therapies, most elegantly and appropriately delivered. Thus, the clinical fantasy I have described here is influenced by neurolinguistics. But a larger influence is also social science—a recognition that language is the major tool that humans have for making and sharing meaning, not an end in itself. Some readers and clinicians might consider this fence-sitting as wishy washy; I prefer to think there is a great view to be seen from this particular fence.

References

Avent, J., Glista, S., Wallace, S., Jackson, J., Nishioka, J., & Yip, W. (2005). Family information needs about aphasia. *Aphasiology, 19,* 365–375.

Beeke, S., Maxim., J., & Wilkinson, R. 2007). Using conversation analysis to assess and treat people with aphasia. In L. Cummings (Ed.), *Pragmatics and adult language disorders, Seminars in Speech and Language, 2,* 136–147.

Bhogal, S., Teasell, R., & Foley, N. (2003). Rehabilitation of aphasia: More is better. *Topics in Stroke Rehabilitation, 10.*

Cherney, L., Halper, A., Holland, A., & Cole, R. (in press). Computerized script training for aphasia: Preliminary results. *American Journal of Speech-Language Pathology.*

Davis, G. A., & Wilcox, M. J., (1985*). Adult aphasia rehabiliation: Applied pragmatics.* San Diego, CA: Singular

Elman, R. (Ed). (2007). *Group treatment of neurogenic communication disorders: The expert clinician's approach.* San Diego, CA: Plural Publishing.

Elman, R., & Bernstein-Ellis, E. (1999). The efficacy of group communication treatment in adults having chronic aphasia: Linguistic and communicative outcome measures. *Journal of Speech, Language and Hearing Research, 42,* 411–419.

Hinckley, J. J., & Craig, H. K. (1998). Influence of rate of treatment on the naming abilities of adults with chronic aphasia. *Aphasiology, 12,* 989–1006.

Holland, A. (2007). *Counseling in communication disorders: A wellness perspective.* San Diego, CA: Plural Publishing.

Holland, A., & Ramage, A. (2004). Learning from Roger Ross: A clinical journey. In J. Duchan & S. Byng (Eds.), *Challenging aphasia therapies.* Hove UK: Psychology Press.

Hopper, T., Holland, A., & Rewega, M. (2002). Conversational coaching: Treatment outcomes and future directions. *Aphasiology, 16,* 745–762.

Kagan, A. (1998). Supported conversation for adult with aphasia: Methods and resources for training conversational partners. *Aphasiology, 12,* 816–830.

Kagan, A., & Gailey, G. (1993). Functional is not enough. Training conversation partners for aphasic adults. In A, Holland& M. Forbes (Eds.), *Aphasia treatment: World perspectives* (pp. 199–225). San Diego: Singular.

Kiran, S., & Thompson, C. (2003). The role of semantic complexity in treatment of naming deficits: Training semantic categories in fluent aphasia by controlling exemplar typicality. *Journal of Speech, Language and Hearing Research, 46,* 608–622.

Maher, L., Kendall, D., Swearengin, J., Rodriguez, A., Leon, M., Pingel, K., et al. (in press) Constraint induced language therapy in chronic aphasia.

Moore, D. (1994). A second start. *Topics in Stroke Rehabilitation,* 1, 100–103.

Parr, S., & Byng, S., (2000). Perspectives and priorities: Accessing user views in functional communication assessment. In L. Worrall & C. M. Frattali (Eds.), *Neurogenic communication disorders: A functional approach.* New York: Thieme.

Pulvermueller, F., Neininger, B., Elbert, T., Mohr, B., Rockstroh, B., Koebbel, P., et al. (2001). Constraint induced therapy of chronic aphasia after stroke. *Stroke, 32,* 16–21.

Quann, E. (2002). *By his side: Life and love after stroke.* Highland MD: Fastrack.

Raymer, A., Beeson, P., Holland, A., Kendall, D., Maher, L., Martin, N., et al. (in press) Translational research in aphasia: From neuroscience to reurorehabilitation. *Journal of Speech, Language and Hearing Research.*

Sarno, M. T., & Peters, J. (2004). *The aphasia handbook, USA edition.* Available through the National Aphasia Association, http://www.aphasia.org.

Shadden, B. (2005). Aphasia as identity theft: Theory and practice. *Aphasiology, 19,* 211–224.

Thompson, C. K. (2007). Complexity in language learning. *American Journal of Speech and Language Pathology, 16,* 3–5.

Thompson, C. K., Shapiro, L., Kiran, S., & Sobecks, J. (2003). The role of syntactic complexity in training wh-movement structures in agrammatic aphasia: The complexity account of treatment efficacy (CATE). *Journal of Speech, Language and Hearing Research, 46,* 591–607.

Worrall, L. E. (1999). *Functional communication therapy planner.* Oxon, UK: Winslow Press.

Worrall, L. E. (2000). The influence of professional values on the functional communication approach in aphasia. In L. E. Worrall & C. M. Frattali (Eds.), *Neurogenic communication disorders: A functional approach.* New York: Thieme.

Youmans, G., Holland, A., Munoz, M., & Bourgeois. (2005). Script training and automaticity in two adults with aphasia. *Aphasiology, 18,* 435–450.

APPENDIX 4A
Selected Internet Resources

Adler Aphasia Center: http://www.Adleraphasiacenter.org

Aphasia Hope Foundation http://www.aphasiahope.org

Aphasia Institute: http://www.aphasia.ca

California Aphasia Center: http://www.Aphasiacenter.org

Connect: http://www.UKConnect.org

National Aphasia Association http://www.aphasia.org

National Stroke Association http://www. stroke.org

Aphasia Help? www.aphasiahelp.org

5

Impairment and Life Consequences Approaches for Fluent Aphasia

Convergences and Divergences

Audrey L. Holland and Anna Basso

This a summary of the ongoing dialogue between Anna Basso and Audrey Holland concerning intervention for MS.

Dr. Basso's View

I like what Dr. Holland suggests, and think that in an ideal world everything should be done. But what she suggests and what I suggest do not seem to me to be alternatives. I think that when Dr. Holland says that you aim to treat the consequences of aphasia, the difference is clear. What I suggest is aimed at helping the patient to reclaim as much as possible of the underlying damaged capacity to process language in the same way as a "normal" person processes language. When a plateau is reached (and this unfortunately almost always happens *before* perfectly restoring language) the *consequences* of aphasia must then be considered and the aphasic person (family, etc.) must be given all possible help in making their best with what is left. This does not mean that the two treatments should be offered in sequence; it means that the rationale underlying them is different.

I think it would help everybody if we understand this difference. It seems to me that the expertise necessary for carrying out the two therapies is different. I am sure that Dr. Holland is very good at her work, but possibly not interested in doing what I do, and not particularly well equipped for doing it.

To sum up, my opinion is that what we offer are two different things. Both are helpful for the patient but defy comparison. In my young days at school, teachers used to say that you cannot add apples and pears. In the same way you cannot compare medical treatment with the psychosocial treatment of aphasia even if both must be instantiated.

Dr. Holland's View

There is literally nothing in Dr. Basso's therapy plan that I object to, and, in fact, I feel certain that MS would profit greatly from the intervention that Dr. Basso proposes. I was surprised to see how her activities for treatment directly applied to MS really were so similar—the stimuli may have varied, but few of the goals varied. Two experienced clinicians, with different theoretical commitments, saw the same problems, both looked to the same positive outcomes. To extend Dr. Basso's analogy, it seemed to me that we are both talking about apples—Dr. Basso is choosing Mackintosh or Golden Delicious, perhaps, and I am choosing Granny Smiths and Northern Spies, but first and foremost, apples are apples.

As I see it, we really part company mostly in our evaluation of clinical roles concerning whether we should move beyond the apples to the pears. "Apples" is language. "Pears" is communication in the real world. I am not sure we differ theoretically. We differ only in where we consider our responsibility to end. And I think that our differences can only energize and move the field forward by offering alternatives for individuals with aphasia and their families in relation to effective treatments.

Finally, I believe Dr. Basso is quite right in suggesting that she and I probably do different things in treatment because we do different things well. For example, I have never been able to keep my sights focused simply on language; I have always been interested in language's role in the larger context of communication. This makes it very likely that my clinical effectiveness is diminished when I concentrate my energies simply on language. I suspect the opposite is true for Dr. Basso. I am sure we both do best what we are most comfortable and enthusiastic about doing.

SECTION III

6

A Case of Severe Apraxia of Speech and Aphasia

David Howard and Nina Simmons-Mackie

Case Description

GJ is a 72-year-old right-handed monolingual Englishman who is aphasic after a major stroke 4 years ago (at the age of 68). He had retired when he was 60 having worked as a farmer, driver, and a mechanic. He left school at the age of 13.

GJ's wife died 6 years ago. His daughter, who is disabled and wheelchair-bound, lives nearby with her daughter and a dog, Titch, who GJ walked daily prior to his stroke. GJ has an electric wheelchair and often goes to visit his daughter and granddaughter. Caregivers come to his home three times a day: to get him up and give him breakfast; to give him lunch; and to get him to bed. His son lives on a remote Scottish island with his family.

GJ is keen on horse racing and can independently go to the betting shop and write out a betting slip. He reads the newspaper every day. His other interests were fishing, car mechanics, and DIY (do-it-yourself home improvements), but he no longer actively pursues these.

He has had a moderate-severe hearing loss all his life and, when he was young, used British Sign Language. A bone-conduction hearing aid was fitted 3 years ago, but he prefers not to use this because of the increased background noise. He is a well-trained and effective lip-reader.

Medical History

GJ had a left middle cerebral artery infarct. This resulted in a severe communication disorder, a dense right hemiplegia, and a right homonymous hemianopia. The hemianopia resolved, but the hemiplegia and communication disorder are still severe. His hearing is impaired, but he is a skilled lip-reader. He wears glasses for reading.

Language

GJ's spoken language is limited to four words: "aye," "no," "why," and "bye," of which only the first two could be used consistently. He supplements this with effective use of gesture. A previous therapist provided him with a communication book consisting mostly of family member names. In addition, he was given a Portacom, a communication device that can say a variety of recorded words and phrases when the buttons are pressed. The words and phrases can be individually chosen and recorded to suit the needs of a client. GJ does not use the communication book or Portacom to augment communication.

GJ feels that his comprehension of spoken language is unimpaired in all contexts, and that he has no difficulty with understanding written language. He finds writing hard, but occasionally writes cards or messages, and can write the names of some of his family members.

Test Results

GJ was administered the following tests to evaluate his speech and language abilities: Pyramids and Palm Trees (Howard & Patterson, 1992), portions of the Comprehensive Aphasia Test (CAT; Swinburn, Porter, & Howard, 2004), portions of the Psycholinguistic Assessment of Language Processing in Aphasia (PALPA; Kay, Lesser, & Coltheart, 1992), a written naming test based on materials developed by Nickels (1995), the New England Pantomime Tests (Duffy & Duffy, 1984) and tests of oral and nonverbal apraxia. The results of these tests are summarized in Table 6–1.

Table 6–1. Aphasia Test scores for GJ

Test	Score	Test	Score
Semantic memory		**Naming**	
Pyramids and Palm Trees Test		CAT naming	0/48
		T score	37
3 picture version (within normal range)	50/52		
Comprehensive Aphasia Test (CAT)		**Reading aloud**	
Semantic memory test	8/10	CAT real word reading	0/48
(T score 47; below normal 5% cutoff)	9/10	T score	38
Spoken language comprehension		**Writing**	
CAT spoken word-to-picture matching	27/30	CAT copying	26/27
		T score	52
(T score 55; above normal 5% cutoff)		(above normal 5% cutoff)	
CAT sentence-picture matching:	22/32	CAT written naming	10/24
		T score	49
(T score 54; below normal 5% cutoff)	(24/32)		
		Written naming of Nickels (1995) items	
Written language comprehension		overall	17/36
CAT written word-to-picture matching	30/30	high frequency	7/18;
		low frequency	10/18

(continues)

Table 6–1. *(continued)*

Test	Score	Test	Score
T score (above normal 5% cutoff)	65	**New England Pantomime Test**	
		Recognition	45/46
		Expression	22/23
Synonym judgments (PALPA 50)	56/60		
(high imageability 28/30; low imageability 28/30; within normal limits)		**Test for oral apraxia**	
		Movements with demonstration	19/19
Repetition		Movements without demonstration	14/19
CAT word repetition	0/35		
T score	35		
CVC words	0/20		
1 syllable	13/20		
2 syllable	2/10		
3 syllable	2/6		

T scores on the CAT have a mean of 50 and a standard deviation of 10 across a large sample of people with aphasia. These scores give information about relative strengths and weaknesses in tests compared with other people with aphasia. Except where stated, GJ's scores are well below normal

Summary of Test Results

For GJ there was no evidence of difficulty in word or sentence comprehension or impairment in semantic memory for either spoken or written language. He was unable to name any items, to repeat, or to read aloud. Written output was better than spoken, but still accurate for less than 50% of picturable items. There was no evidence of apraxia for nonverbal oral movements, although GJ found repetition and voluntary production of both speech sounds and words either extremely difficult or impossible.

In short, GJ's spoken output is limited by a severe articulatory apraxia (not affecting nonspeech oral movements). This results in almost complete failure in any task requiring spoken production. Written naming is poor, but much better than spoken production.

Gesture is good in both comprehension and production. Language comprehension, for both spoken and written language, is relatively good.

References

Duffy, R. J., & Duffy, J. R. (1984). *New England Pantomime Tests.* Austin, TX: Pro-Ed.

Howard, D., & Patterson, K. (1992). *The Pyramids and Palm Trees test: A test of semantic access from words and pictures.* Bury St. Edmunds, UK: Thames Valley Test Company.

Nickels, L. A. (1995). Getting it right—Using aphasic naming errors to evaluate theoretical models of spoken word recognition. *Language and Cognitive Processes, 10*(1), 13–45.

Kay, J., Lesser, R., & Coltheart, M. (1992) *Psycholinguistic Assessments of Language Processing in Aphasia.* New York: Psychology Press.

Swinburn, K., Porter, G., & Howard, D. (2004). *Comprehensive Aphasia Test.* Hove, UK: Psychology Press.

7

Intervention for a Case of Severe Apraxia of Speech and Aphasia: A Functional-Social Perspective

Nina Simmons-Mackie

Introduction

Intervention for GJ is rooted in approaches that aim to maximize life with communication disability. Biopsychosocial models of health and social models of disability provide useful frameworks in this regard. Biopsychosocial models define disability in terms of an interaction between an individual's personal attributes, abilities or impairments and barriers or supports within the environment. Thus, disability is associated with both internal and external factors (World Health Organization, 2001). Social models stress the creation of disability by barriers in the environment and the impact of society on functioning and disability (Finkelstein, 1991; Fougeyrollas, Noreau, Bergeron, Cloutier, Dion, & St-Michel, 1998; Oliver, 1996).

In addition, intervention principles specific to aphasia such as the Life Participation Approach to Aphasia (LPAA, 2000, 2001) and functional-social approaches to aphasia and related disorders (e.g., Byng & Duchan, 2005; Duchan, 2001; Elman, 2005; Holland, 1982; Pound, Parr, Lindsay, & Woolf, 2000; Sarno, 2004; Simmons-Mackie, 1988, 1998a, 1998b, 2000, 2001a, 2001b; Simmons-Mackie & Damico, 1995, 1996b; Worrall, 2000) guide intervention for GJ. LPAA sets forth specific guidelines for management of aphasia as follows: (1) the explicit goal of intervention is enhancement of life participation, (2) all those affected are entitled to services, (3) measures of success include documented life enhancement, (4) both personal and environmental factors are targets of intervention, and (5) emphasis is on availability of services as needed at all stages. Others have provided philosophical frameworks and explicit intervention methods for implementing functional-social approaches (e.g. Pound et al, 2000; Simmons-Mackie, 1998a, 1998b, 2000, 2001a, 2001b). Suggestions for implementing a functional-social approach are offered as follows: (1) address both information exchange and social needs as dual goals of communication; (2) address communication needs within authentic, relevant, and natural contexts; (3) view communication as dynamic, flexible, and multidimensional; (4) focus on the collaborative nature of communication; (5) focus on natural discourse genres such as conversation; (6) focus on the consequences of aphasia; (7) focus on adaptations to impairment; and (8) embrace the perspective of those affected by aphasia (Simmons-Mackie, 2000, 2001a, 2001b). Functional-social approaches are designed to promote membership in a communicating society and participation in personally relevant activities by reducing communication disability. The approaches are consumer driven and client centered. Client-centered practice involves collecting information from the client to assess functioning and participation, focusing outcome targets on the life situations that are important to the client and ensuring client choice and decision-making in therapy. Finally, functional-social approaches focus on identity and psychosocial function as inherent elements of communication.

GJ's intervention is also guided by Living with Aphasia: Framework for Outcome Measurement (A-FROM; Kagan, Simmons-Mackie, Rowland, Huijbregts, Shumway, McEwen, et al., in press). This conceptual model was designed to guide intervention and outcome targets for persons living with aphasia. It is an adaptation of the

World Health Organization's International Classification of Functioning, Disability and Health (WHO ICF) (WHO, 2001). Based on A-FROM the clincan and GJ would explore five domains including: (1) satisfaction with life with aphasia/apraxia of speech (e.g., well-being and quality of life), (2) participation in home and community, (3) barriers or facilitators to communication and participation, (4) personal factors such as identity and feelings related to aphasia, and (5) severity and pattern of communication deficits (i.e., impairments). These domains constitute the framework delineated in Figure 7-1.

Although adapted from the WHO ICF, A-FROM highlights the dynamic interaction among domains and the overlap of domains that constitute quality of life at the center. In addition, this framework expands the notion of personal factors to include aspects such as identity, confidence, and feelings—important components of communicative engagement. In keeping with these models and

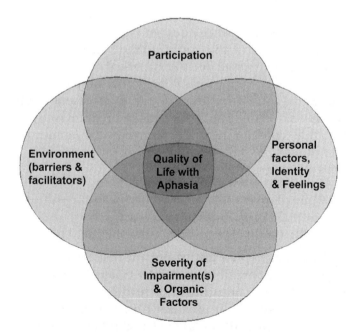

Figure 7–1. Living with aphasia: Framework for Outcome Measurement (A-FROM). (Adapted with permission of the Aphasia Institute, Toronto, Canada.)

principles, intervention for GJ includes a focus on reducing deficits, improving participation, maximizing environmental support, and enhancing personal identity and overall quality of life.

Case Interpretation

GJ presents with severe apraxia of speech (AOS) and aphasia. Memory and general attention have been deemed functionally intact. In spite of right hemiplegia, GJ is healthy and mobile with an electric wheelchair. He dropped out of school at age 13, but was literate prior to his stroke 4 years ago. Presently expressive communication is limited to four words, gesture, body language, and efforts to write words. His attempts to communicate with family and caregivers often result in unresolved breakdowns. Although he was given an electronic communication device ("Portacom") and a communication book, GJ does not use these. His activities include visiting his daughter, reading the newspaper, and placing bets on horse races. He lives alone, rarely sees old friends, and avoids engaging in communication with people he does not know. Although he is able to leave his home, visit family, and go to the betting shop, he feels bored, lonely, and depressed due to his marked communication difficulty and social isolation. GJ has come to our outpatient clinic to participate in an aphasia program due to dissatisfaction with his current functional status. The mission of the program is to enhance communication skills, to maximize life with communication disability, and promote psychosocial well-being for people affected by aphasia and related disorders.

Additional Assessment

Based on the results of prior testing at a university clinic, GJ was diagnosed with severe apraxia of speech (AOS) and moderate expressive aphasia with mild impairment of reading and auditory comprehension. This assessment provides a baseline inventory of GJ's language impairment and motor speech abilities. Further assessment is needed to determine GJ's use of communication in relevant environments and his current and desired level of participation in communicative events and life situations. Figure 7–2 presents the A-

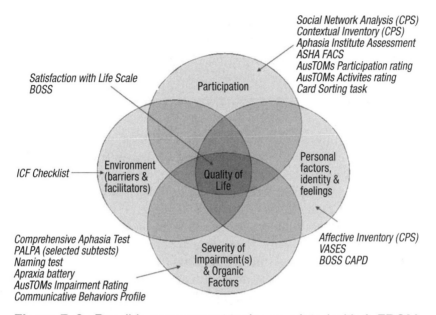

Figure 7–2. Possible assessment tools associated with A-FROM domains.

FROM model with the relevant assessment tools that have been or might be used in GJ's assessment, and are described below.

Assessment of Multiple Domains

Several approaches to assessment are used to capture multiple domains including impairment, participation, personal factors, environmental factors, and overall well-being. Assessment includes both qualitative and quantitative methods.

A qualitative assessment is conducted to gain insight into GJ's communicative life and functional communication. This data collection strategy draws from qualitative assessment including the Communicative Profiling System (CPS; Simmons-Mackie & Damico, 1996a, 2001a, 2001b). The CPS was designed to identify key features associated with communication in a person's everyday life. Several qualitative data collection strategies are used including interview, observation and self-report via journaling (with the help of caretakers and family if needed). Data are collected using four "profiles" including (1) a contextual profile describing relevant contexts of communication (e.g., life situations, roles, activities), (2) a social network profile that describes relevant people and relationships, (3) a behavioral profile that includes communicative behaviors, barriers, strategies, and resources used, and (4) an affective profile describing feelings regarding communication and life with communication disability.

Ethnographic interviewing is an important element of this qualitative assessment.[1] Interviews including GJ, family members, and/ or caregivers would be consistent with an open-ended, ethnographic style to gather personal perspectives and priorities (see Spradley, 1979; Westby, 1990, Westby, Burda, & Mehta, 2003). The aphasia literature suggests that interview and observation are excellent methods of collecting authentic data for goal setting, intervention planning, and outcome assessment (e.g., Davidson, Worrall, & Hickson, 2006; Parr & Byng, 2000; Simmons-Mackie & Damico, 1996, 2001a, 2001b). Moreover, self-report is a critical element of measuring participation and personal factors (Cruice, Worrall, Hickson, & Murison, 2005). Research suggests that people with aphasia are capable of reliable self-report, and self-report tends to differ from proxy reports particularly regarding communication and emotional factors (Cruice et al., 2005; Doyle, 2005; Eadie, Yorkston, Klasner, Dudgeon, Deitz, Baylor, et al., 2006; Hafsteinsdotter & Grypdonck, 1997; Lomas, Pickard, & Mohide, 1987). Initially the interview would be aimed at "getting to know" GJ as a person—his likes and dislikes, aspirations, and life experiences. Because of his severe expressive difficulties, a variety of conversational supports (e.g., maps, written supports, drawing, gestures, photographs, pictographs) would be employed to ensure that he has a means of expressing his ideas (e.g., Kagan, Winckel, & Shumway, 1996). The efficacy of supported communication (e.g., "Supported Conversation" [SCA™]) has been demonstrated (Kagan, Black, Duchan, Simmons-Mackie, & Square, 2001). In addition to getting a feel for the person behind the communication disability, the interview would focus on identifying GJ's communicative strengths, relevant communication contexts, activi-

---

[1]Ethnographic interviews tend to be open-ended and follow the lead of the person being interviewed in order to capture his or her perspectives (in contrast to structured, interviewer-controlled questions devised a priori). See Westby (1990) or Spradley (1979) for descriptions.

ties, and partners as described in the frameworks above. For example, during the interview GJ might be asked about who he sees and what he does in a typical week. They might discuss barriers to communication and useful strategies. The interview would also include a discussion of potential goals. For example, he may be asked: "in 6 months what would you like to be doing differently in your life?" Again a variety of resources and supports would be employed to allow GJ to express himself. Interview strands might focus on particular activities of interest to GJ. This focus on communication in context orients the person to think beyond the obvious goal of "talking," to the functional goal of communicating "for what purposes." In addition, GJ's comfort and skill with various supported communication resources would be explored to help identify potential strategies and resources. Thus, intervention would be designed to address the unique life consequences of GJ's communication disability. The interview would address the consequences of aphasia, AOS, and hearing loss as well as other issues affecting GJ's communicative life (e.g., mobility). Although the initial interview is an important baseline, the interview and goal-setting process are dynamic and evolutionary. Thus, the clinician and GJ would have an ongoing dialogue to flesh out potential outcome targets and variables that might influence real-life outcomes as intervention proceeds.

In addition to interviewing, observational data will provide information about actual communication. The client and caregivers will be instructed in use of a small video camera to be taken home to videotape social interactions within relevant settings (e.g., home with caregiver, visiting with daughter). Such videotapes provide valuable information on "real life" communication that might not be apparent during clinical interactions or interviews. Using videotapes the clinician might conduct discourse analyses to identify GJ's communicative strengths and problems as well as those of his usual communication partners (e.g., Boles, 1998; Booth & Perkins, 1999; Lock, Wilkinson, Bryan, Maxim, Edmundson, & Bruce, 2001; Oelschlaeger & Damico, 2000; Simmons-Mackie & Kagan, 1999). For example, methods of repair can be studied to determine if intervention might provide more efficient or effective repair strategies with particular partners. The results of qualitative data collection and discourse analyses will provide data in all key domains of A-FROM including participation, impairment, personal factors, environmental factors, and overall quality of life.

In addition, quantitative analysis of communicative behaviors can be conducted via discourse analysis (e.g., number of repairs, variety of speech acts, information units). Quantitative results can also be gleaned from other outcome measures such as the Australian Therapy Outcome Measures (AusTOMs; Perry, Morris, Unsworth, Duckett, Skeat, Dodd, et al., 2004). The AusTOMs allow clinicians to rate the areas of language, speech, cognitive-communication, swallowing, and fluency across four domains (impairment, activity, participation, and overall well-being) using a 0 to 5 scale. Psychometric properties of the tool have been demonstrated (Morris, Perry, Unsworth, Skeat, Taylor, Dodd, et al., 2005; Unsworth, Duckett, Duncombe, Perry, Skeat, & Taylor, 2004).

Assessment of Impairment

No further formal testing specifically targeting GJ's language, cognitive, or motor speech deficits are conducted as baseline measures are available. However, discourse analysis and qualitative assessment provide additional data regarding his impairments, as well as his own estimation of his impairments and strengths. In addition, a baseline measure of writing tasks is collected to more clearly understand his written expression problems and abilities. Comparison of written and spoken word findings also provide more information on the relative contribution of motor versus linguistic deficits. Further analysis might be conducted to determine the source of aphasic expressive deficits (e.g., phonological, semantic) to aid in identifying potential strategies to facilitate expressive language.

As GJ has a moderate-severe hearing loss and has not been using hearing aids due to interference of background noise, an audiologic assessment will be available to determine if there are options for improved function. In addition, if GJ so chooses he will be referred to other rehabilitation team members to assess his potential for improved mobility and performance of activities of daily living. In addition, medical referral for depression might be indicated for GJ.

Assessment of Participation and Activities

Participation includes one's life roles and habits such as managing finances, maintaining relationships, fulfilling job duties, or participating in leisure activities. A *contextual/participation inventory* is completed to identify GJ's key activities and roles prior to onset and at present (Table 7–1) and a *social network profile* will visibly depict GJ's ongoing and regular relationships (Figure 7–3) (from the *CPS*, Simmons-Mackie & Damico, 1996a, 2001a, 2001b). The data for these profiles come from the interviews and observations described above.

In addition, the participation questions of the Aphasia Institute Assessment (AIA)[2] would be administered (Kagan, Simmons-Mackie, Rowland, Huijbregts, Shumway, McEwen et al., unpublished). This "aphasia friendly" tool allows GJ to rate on a 9-point scale whether he is participating as much as he wishes in the areas of roles and responsibilities (e.g., finances, home management), relationships, conversation, and activities such as leisure and recreation. The tool is currently being piloted to assess its psychometric properties. In addition, GJ will indicate on rating scales if "aphasia" is the barrier to participation. Figure 7–4 presents one example of

Table 7–1. GJ's Major Activities Prior to the Onset of Aphasia and at the Time of the Interview

Preonset Activities	Postonset Activities
Visiting family	Visiting daughter
Walking dog (Titch)	
Reading newspaper	Reading newspaper
Fishing	
Car repair	
Carpentry and home repair	
Going to horse races and betting	Going to betting shop
Visiting the pub	

---

[2]The AIA is based on A-FROM and provides ratings in all domains including severity of impairment, participation, environmental factors, personal/emotional factors, and overall quality of life with aphasia.

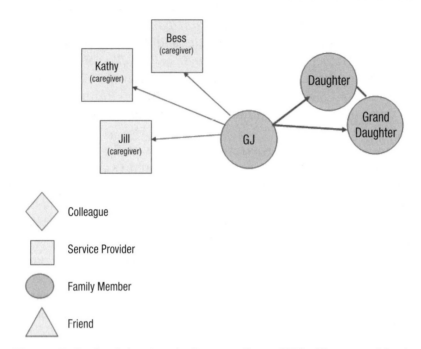

Figure 7–3. Social network diagram (from CPS, Simmons-Mackie & Damico, 2001a) representing people with whom GJ regularly interacts after the onset of aphasia but before functional-social intervention.

the graphics and rating scale of the AIA. Card sorting tasks might also be used to determine activities and life situations that GJ engages in now, used to engage in, or never engaged in (Haley, Jenkins, Hadden, Womack, Hall, & Schweiker, 2005; Simmons-Mackie, 2000, 2001). All of these approaches provide valuable information on life with aphasia and could serve as baselines for future outcome comparisons. Finally, the ASHA Functional Assessment of Communication Skills (ASHA FACS) (Frattali, Thompson, Holland, Wohl, & Ferketic, 1995) might be completed to determine daily tasks that GJ currently performs and his level of performance. Again data for rating performance will derive from interviews and observation. It is possible that intervention could improve his functional status and reduce his dependence on caregivers if GJ wishes.

Finances and Money

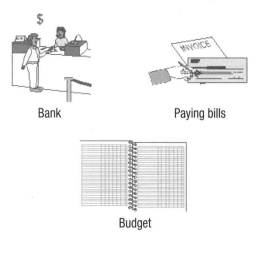

Bank   Paying bills

Budget

Are you doing as much as you want?

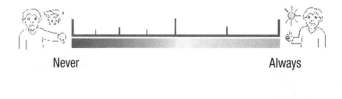

Never   Always

Figure 7–4. Example of a question pertaining to participation in management of personal finances from the Aphasia Institute Assessment (AIA) (Kagan et al., unpublished. Printed with permission from the Aphasia Institute, Toronto, Canada).

Assessment of Environmental Factors

A growing literature documents the impact of the environment on communication disability (e.g., Worrall, Rose, Howe, McKenna, & Hickson, 2007). Therefore, based on interviews and observations, barriers and facilitators to GJ's communication and participation within relevant environments are documented via a checklist adapted from the WHO ICF list of environmental factors (WHO, 2001).

Assessment of Personal Factors and Subjective Well-Being

Communication disability potentially has significant effects on one's emotional well-being, confidence and personal identity (Astrom, Asplund, & Astrom, 1992; Brumfitt, 1993; Muller, 1999; Sarno, 2004; Shadden, 2005). Frequent communicative failures contribute to increased social isolation and a negative sense of self. As GJ has identified loneliness, boredom, and depression as factors influencing his desire for therapy, it is important to document baseline affective levels that might change with intervention. Tools that might be used to document GJ's emotional well-being include the Visual Analogue Self-Esteem Scale (VASES; Brumfitt & Sheeran, 1999), Affect Balance Scale (Bradburn, 1969), the BOSS Communication-Associated Psychological Distress Scale (BOSS CAPD; Doyle, McNeil, Hula, & Mikolic, 2003) or the Satisfaction with Life Scale (SWLS; Diener, Emmons, Larsen, & Griffin, 1985).

Treatment Goals

Treatment planning is a collaborative process with the client assuming a significant role in decision-making. As GJ has severe expressive problems, the SLP is required to possess significant skill in supported conversation to ensure collaborative treatment planning. The SLP prepares appropriate "support" resources for a goal conference. Together the SLP and GJ would select goals, list the needed resources, and identify people available to help achieve potential goals. With the clinician sharing information about potential treatment approaches and the client sharing information about desired plans and outcomes, the clinician and client can arrive at the preferred goals and treatment approach. Following are hypothetical examples of goals that GJ might select:

1. Improve communication of needs and desires to caregivers,
2. Improve conversations with caregivers at home, with daughter and granddaughter, and with friends or acquaintances,
3. Increase communication with son and grandchildren who live in Scotland,

4. Improve management of emergencies at home or in the community,
5. Increase communication and social participation beyond caregivers and immediate family,
6. Improve performance of functional everyday writing tasks (e.g., lists, messages),
7. Increase participation in self-care and home responsibilities.

Once general goals are identified the clinician and GJ would prioritize goals, discuss how the goals might be accomplished, and arrive at any necessary subcomponents of targeted goals. Based on these discussions, individual Goal Attainment Scales (GAS) (Schlosser, 2004) would be devised as one means of measuring progress. GAS are personally relevant 5-point scales developed to "grade" attainment of an overall goal or functional component of a goal. When properly devised, these rating scales have "known" psychometric properties that allow outcomes to be aggregated across goals (Schlosser, 2004). For example, the following scale might be relevant for measuring a subcomponent of goal three above—communicating with his son:

0 Independently e-mails son with no difficulty
1 Independently e-mails son with difficulty
2 E-mails son using "cheat sheet" supports
3 Emails son with caregiver assistance
4 Does not e-mail son

Treatment

GJ appears to be a good candidate for functional intervention because he is highly motivated to improve his functional status and life participation, has relatively good comprehension in spite of restricted speech and writing, has access to the community via an electric powered wheelchair and disability transport, is in good health, and has the support of caregivers and family. Furthermore, his 4 years of living with a communication disability provide GJ with a valuable experiential perspective that will help him evaluate goals for enhancing quality of life. Assuming that GJ would so choose, he will be scheduled for both individual and group therapy for aphasia/AOS. Individual therapy will focus on specific communicative goals and guided practice, whereas group therapy will provide a supportive context for implementing communicative strategies and building communicative confidence. It should be noted that the interventions are described under the domain headings of multiple domains, participation, environment, personal factors, and impairment. For some of the interventions this division is arbitrary as the interventions involve other domains. Therefore, the headings refer to the most obvious intervention activity, not necessarily the domain that is affected by the intervention. For example, participation intervention could require changes in the environment. Moreover, working on participating in a leisure activity might help alleviate GJ's boredom and depression.

Intervention Targeting Multiple Domains

GJ will be enrolled in group conversation therapy designed to (1) provide opportunities for participation in successful conversation, (2) provide supported practice of communication strategies, (3) provide education regarding stroke and community resources, and (4) bolster communicative confidence and positive identity. Studies suggest that well-managed group therapy practiced within a functional-social approach differs significantly from traditional, therapist-centered, impairment-oriented groups in targets of intervention, interactive patterns, discourse sequences, and clinician management style (Kovarsky, Kimbarrow, & Kastner, 1999; Simmons-Mackie, Elman, Holland, & Damico, 2007). Group interaction within a functional-social approach tends toward egalitarian discourse patterns and a client-centered focus. The interaction among participants, rather than therapist feedback and instruction, is the key to successful group therapy. GJ will join an existing group of four people with aphasia who range from very severe to mild-moderate aphasia. Assuming that GJ is interested in this approach, GJ might work on verbal production in context, flexible use of various strategies to augment verbal communication, and methods to repair communicative breakdowns. During group discussion GJ would also learn about stroke and aphasia, about community resources, and about opportunities for community participation. Another significant element of the group context is the opportunity to build self-confidence and shape a positive sense of self. For example, using pictures and props GJ might be recruited to offer advice to group members about car maintenance and repair (prior to onset he was a mechanic and enjoyed auto repair). Similarly, GJ's familiarity with the news and the availability of newspapers and magazines will provide GJ with a means of demonstrating his knowledge of current events. Opportunities to show "what you know" and "who you are" constitute strong influences on a robust sense of self. In addition, the group leader understands group process and counseling allowing participants to explore feelings, and support one another. A randomized controlled trial of group therapy for aphasia based on a functional-social approach demonstrated significant gains on standard language batteries as well as positive psychosocial outcomes for individuals with chronic aphasia (Elman & Bernstein-Ellis, 1999a, 1999b).

Intervention Targeting Impairment

As severe AOS appears to be the most significant barrier to GJ's expressive communication, Sound Production Training (SPT) would be initiated to reduce the expressive impairment. This AOS treatment is designed to improve production of selected target sounds in syllables, words, or phrases using modeling, imitation, integral stimulation, articulatory placement, and production cuing (Wambaugh, 2001). Minimal contrast pairs would be used to differentiate sounds and words. GJ's stimulability to production of various CVs and CVCs is tested to determine initial therapy targets. In addition, his automatic productions (aye, bye, why, and no) might serve as starting points if perseveration can be controlled. To aid generalization of training, functional targets would be selected in sound production training. For example, simple key words or phrases from scripts (see below) might be included in SPT. Thus, GJ might be able to combine speech productions (or approximations) and other modes to express himself and give the "feel" of spoken communication. In a review of research evidence supporting SPT, Wambaugh (2001) notes that this intervention has been systematically investigated for AOS coexisting with aphasia, and can result in improved productions of target sounds. Moreover, "training relatively few exemplars results in improved production of untrained exemplars" (Wambaugh, 2001, p. 12). Potential limitations to the training would be GJ's aphasic word-finding problems and the severity of his AOS.

Interventions Targeting Participation

Ross and Wertz (2003, p. 355) studied quality of life after aphasia and concluded that "therapy that focuses on situation-specific communication and societal participation appears to be most appropriate for enhancing QOL of people with chronic aphasia." Level of participation is more highly correlated with positive QOL than performance of daily activities or severity of impairment (Eadie et al., 2006). In addition, a robust social network has been equated with improved quality of life and life satisfaction after stroke (Anderson & Fridlund, 2002; Astrom et al., 1992), and the number and quality of social relationships and events influence opportunities for communication. GJ currently lacks a wide choice of communicative partners and he participates in relatively few communicative situations. His daily activities (reading the newspaper and placing bets) do not afford rich and varied communication opportunities. As improved language or communication do not automatically enhance life participation, an array of interventions might focus directly on increasing GJ's participation in specific life situations and on increasing the variety of communication partners. This activity related intervention involves identifying roles, events, or activities in which GJ would like to participate and facilitating participation by altering the environment, training partners, and/or teaching GJ strategies for achieving participation (Simmons-Mackie, 2000, 2001a). For example, GJ might like to expand his betting activities to involve attendance at horse races with a selected group of friends or watching races at a neighborhood pub. If a suitable volunteer could be included in partner training (see below), then this volunteer could facilitate GJ's reintegration into such an event (Lyon, 1996; Lyon, Carisk, Keisler, Rosenbek, Levine, Kumpula et al., 1997). The SLP would serve as a consultant, identifying potential communicative barriers to participation and helping GJ brainstorm and implement possible remedies. One key to this approach is the need for the SLP to maximize the potential for success; a failed re-entry attempt tends to decrease confidence and further reinforce a sense of social isolation.

Various communication resources and strategies could facilitate GJ's participation in events. Thus, GJ and the SLP collaboratively identify and implement a host of communication resources and strategies to enhance communication including augmentative and alternative communication (AAC) options and conversational management strategies. AAC options are particularly appropriate due to GJ's severe AOS. In a review of the literature on augmentative and alternative communication (AAC) and AOS, Rogers (2001, p. 27) suggests that "individuals with AOS have great potential to benefit from AAC . . ." and aphasic deficits "should not preclude these individuals from using AAC." Based on published guidelines, AAC options should involve multiple modes of communicating and tap into GJ's full range of communication abilities (National Joint Committee for the Communication Needs of Persons with Severe Disabilities, 1992). Resources might include communication books (e.g., organized pictures and/or written words), electronic communication devices, graphics such as maps or pictographs, or remnant books (scrapbook of "remnants" such as newspaper clippings, movie ticket stub, menu). Various augmentative strategies would be explored such as drawing, pointing to letters or written displays, writing words, phrases, or parts of words, gesture, pantomime, and other means of augmenting residual speech or vocalizations. In addition to "transactional" strategies designed to communicate information, therapy for GJ would also focus on skill in managing social discourse (Simmons-Mackie & Damico, 1995, 1996b). For example, GJ might improve his ability to employ interactional strategies such as layering communicative modes, using affiliative moves and engagement strategies, shifting the communicative burden to a partner, referencing shared information, or building on partner utterances (see Goodwin, 1995; Simmons-Mackie, Kingston, & Schultz, 2005). Other strategies such as self-cues to word retrieval or phoneme selection and sequencing self-cues during conversation would be tailored to GJ's linguistic and motor impairments. In addition to general options, resources specific to various needs might be useful such as creating audio recordings for emergency calls, developing caregiver instruction checklists, or developing "cheat sheets" for written tasks (e.g., standard messages to friends, shopping lists). Particular communicative functions would be identified to incorporate into GJ's communication. For example, GJ feels a loss at his inability to tell jokes; intervention might involve alternative means of expressing his sense of humor (e.g., cartoons, written jokes, drawing) (Simmons-Mackie, 2004).

GJ and the SLP would assess his current use of resources and strategies. For example, GJ has not used the Portacom provided by a prior therapist; nor has he used his communication book. Barriers to use of these options would be explored and if appropriate, modifications and situated training implemented. Garrett and Beukelman (1998) suggest that clients should learn how to flexibly use a variety of communicative options and these should be integrated into everyday situations. In fact, failure to train in natural situations is one of the most common reasons for AAC failure (Bellaire, Beorges, & Thompson, 1991; Garrett & Beukelman, 1998). In addition, user satisfaction with AAC is an important element in ongoing use. AAC can call attention to the person as disabled, disrupt or slow down the social interaction, or actually fail to enhance communication. If an approach is not efficient, effective, or valued, then it is unlikely that it will be used (Rogers, 2001). Drawing from Rogers (2001), the following guidelines may be implemented, if GJ desires, to promote flexible, multimodal communication including a variety of options that suit his everyday needs: (1) GJ's individual abilities and needs will drive his AAC options, (2) selected vocabulary for AAC training will reflect GJ's real life needs, (3) GJ will engage in simulated and real life-practice using AAC, and (4) training of communicative partners will be integrated into AAC training. The ultimate objective will be to build GJ's use of multimodal communication and his skill in managing the give and take of everyday communicative interactions.

As GJ engages in several routine encounters, participation in these events might be improved through conversational coaching, script training, or situation-specific training. These treatments have been offered as methods of practicing "ritualized" or preplanned interactions to meet specific communication needs of people with aphasia (Hopper & Holland, 1998; Hopper, Holland, & Rewega, 2002; Youmans, Holland, & Munoz, 2005). Although we typically think of scripts as "spoken" interactions, scripts for GJ would employ multimodal communication due to his limited verbal expression. Scripts would be developed for regular scenarios occurring in GJ's life. For example, GJ might learn scripts for instructing daily caregivers, making meal selections, instructing a transport driver, or making an emergency phone call. Scripts, developed in conjunction with GJ, would include various communication modes and resources to supplement GJ's limited speech. For example, regular caregiver instructions might involve scripts with specific checklists, preselected pictographs, written words, gestures, or selections on a communication device. These scripts or scenarios would be practiced within therapy with the clinician and then with other partners to ensure that the targeted communicative objective is realized. It is anticipated that richly contextualized script practice would aid generalization of communication strategies to other communicative events.

Due to his relatively good reading comprehension, GJ is a candidate for learning to negotiate the Internet and use electronic mail. Therefore, GJ will be instructed in basic computer skills, negotiating the Internet, and using e-mail (including left-handed typing). This will expand his opportunities to communicate with his son, grandchildren, and friends, and obtain information and entertainment via the Internet. A local charity that provides computers to disabled individuals will provide the needed hardware and software. Computer instruction is available in the speech and hearing clinic where volunteers teach basic computer skills to clients. Although GJ has marked difficulty writing, he can recognize written target words and write fragments of words. Therefore, he might profit from learning spell check and dictionary/thesaurus options to aid written/typed composition via computer. Home assignments might include writing e-mail messages to his clinician or his son in Scotland or "looking for" specific information on the Internet (e.g., information about aphasia, find jokes to share with aphasia group). A "peer mentor" (a member of the aphasia group) who is skilled in using the Internet will be available to provide ongoing assistance to GJ as needed. This intervention will not only expand GJ's social network and participation via the Internet, but also might improve his functional communication and writing.

As GJ enjoys reading the newspaper, he might enjoy joining an aphasia book club. This reading intervention program revolves around the concept of a typical adult book club in which participants choose a book and read segments to discuss in weekly meetings. Unlike standard book clubs, the aphasia book club provides reading supports and materials graded to individual reading abilities. Thus, an adult reading experience is nested within a carefully programmed therapy approach. Plans and materials for aphasia book clubs have been developed and field tested by Bernstein-Ellis and Elman (2006, 2007). Not only does this reading program increase participation in a leisure activity, but also the program might improve reading skill, provide opportunities for social interaction, and improve written expression.

Also, during the course of therapy other interests may be explored. For example, once GJ is comfortable in the group therapy situation, he might like to join the aphasia advocacy program. Members identify and implement various plans for promoting greater awareness and understanding of aphasia. For example, group members have formed an aphasia speaker's bureau. Speaker's bureau members provide presentations to the community. For example, they speak to newly enrolled nursing students at a local university. Each member with aphasia presents a "story" of a personal experience with health care to sensitize nurses to issues in health care that affect people with aphasia (e.g., decision-making, being treated as incompetent). Although the SLP is not involved in the advocacy program, the SLP might help GJ devise a script and supports for a presentation. For example, GJ might choose to use PowerPoint slides supplemented with preprogrammed phrases "spoken" by his Portacom, props, spoken exclamations, and gestures to tell his story. In addition to advocacy and political action, this sort of activity reinforces the utility of "total" communication approaches, instills confidence and pride, and fosters a strong group identity.

As GJ becomes more familiar with the aphasia program, he might choose to become more active in various consumer-oriented projects. For example, he might wish to join the consumer board that conducts annual program evaluation of the clinic, or he might participate in a rehabilitation program committee (e.g., safety, fundraising, research). Such activities provide participation opportunities and, more importantly, represent the administration's belief in shared planning and consumer input at all levels.

Intervention Targeting the Environment

As effective communication does not depend on GJ's skills alone, communication partner training would be an appropriate target of intervention. Partner communicative skill, knowledge, and attitude are important components of the communicative environment for people with communication disabilities. There is a growing literature describing various approaches to improving communication by including family, friends, or volunteer partners in therapy (Avent & Austermann, 2003; Boles, 1997, 1998; Booth & Perkins, 1999; Cranfill, Simmons-Mackie, & Kearns, 2005; Garrett & Beukelman, 1995; Hickey, Olswang, & Bourgeois, 2004; Hinckley & Packard, 2001; Ho, Weiss, Garrett, & Lloyd, 2005; Kagan & Gailey, 1993; Lyon et al., 1997; Purdy & Hindenlang, 2005; Rayner & Marshall, 2003 Simmons-Mackie, Kearns, & Potechin, 1987/2005; Sorin-Peters, 2004). Approaches include behavioral training to alter communication patterns, counseling approaches, and adult education formats involving individual partners, dyads or groups. A randomized controlled trial demonstrated that trained volunteers scored significantly higher than untrained volunteers in communicating with people with aphasia. Training also resulted in positive change in the ratings of people with aphasia even though these individuals did not participate in training (Kagan, Black, Duchan, Simmons-Mackie, & Square, 2001). The goal of partner training is to create skilled partners who support and facilitate communication. Communication resources and strategies discussed above can be employed by communication partners, and partners can learn how to support an enjoyable communicative interaction. Potential partners could be identified from the social network analysis. In the case of GJ, his daughter and selected caregivers in the home might be included in intervention. Once trained, these partners would be able to train other partners to facilitate total communication. This intervention would be designed to build enjoyment and success of conversation and related genres. In addition, participation oriented intervention would include attention to reducing environmental barriers and increasing communicative access for GJ (Lubinski, 2001; Worrall, Rose, Howe, McKenna, & Hickson, 2007). Family members would also be invited to attend a family support group where they can share experiences and expand their knowledge of aphasia and related topics.

Intervention Focusing on Identity and Emotional Factors

Attention to identity development and self-concept is an integral part of intervention with GJ as communication disabilities can affect identity and self-concept (Herrmann & Wallesch, 1989; Sarno,

2004; Shadden, 2005; Simmons-Mackie, 2000, 2001). Research has demonstrated that communication ability can predict psychological well-being and social health, and emotional health strongly influences social participation (Cruice, Worrall, Hickson, & Murison, 2003). In a social approach any intervention activity must integrate methods that foster a robust sense of self. Thus, most of the intervention options discussed above include an element of "person-centered" management and counseling style that are actively designed to promote feelings, of autonomy, self-worth, and positive identity. However, it is possible to program activities that explicitly focus on exploring identity and maximizing affective well-being. For example, the SLP might suggest activities that involve exploring life with communication disability such as keeping a journal. Journaling involves keeping notes on some topic such as daily activities, feelings or observations. Using a structured "template" provided by the SLP, GJ can document "daily life" by making multimodal "entries" such as writing, drawings, remnants (e.g., clip from TV guide, computer printout), comments by others, or photos taken with his digital camera. The journal provides insight into life with communication disability and serves as a way to explore "who I am" since the onset of aphasia/AOS. Also, a journal serves as a context for initiating conversations (possibly in the aphasia group) and provides experience in generating propositions through multiple modes.

Time Management in a Functional-Social Approach

The preceding list of potential interventions is long. One might wonder how much time would be consumed by such a rich array of treatments. In fact, there is considerable overlap in the approaches and programs established within this philosophy and parallel services are often funded in various ways and managed in a variety of formats (e.g., volunteers, family, self-help). For example, the aphasia book club would be a separate service funded through a per "book" fee that is distinct from individual or group therapy (Bernstein-Ellis & Elman, 2006, 2007). Computer and Internet training would be managed by volunteers who are trained for this purpose. Although the SLP might help GJ with a presentation for the speaker's bureau, the aphasia advocacy program and speaker's bureau are run by people with aphasia and their families. Thus, the role of the SLP in many of these services or programs is consultative. The SLP would be directly responsible for managing group therapy and carrying out Sound Production, AAC, script, and partner training. The latter three therapy activities might be integrated to be targeted simultaneously. Volunteers and caregivers/family members would be recruited to help fabricate resources, assist with home practice, or expand the circle of partners trained. For activity specific intervention the SLP might work with GJ and a communication partner or volunteer who then participate in the activity and report back to the SLP. Thus, the SLP need not commit significant time to attending various community events. In other words, once a functional-social philosophy is integrated into an organization, then the entire program can be developed to support multiple facets of intervention.

Team Management

In addition to speech-language pathology, other services will be available to GJ such as audiology/aural rehabilitation, physical therapy, and occupational therapy. If GJ chooses to take advantage of these services, then goals and intervention plans may be integrated across therapies to maximize functional outcome. Also, GJ and his caregivers may be introduced to a range of resources such as local stroke support groups, National Aphasia Association, Aphasia Hope Foundation, and other sources.

Outcome Measures

The models and data collection methods that guided assessment of GJ will also guide outcome measurement. It is important that assessment include the domains of impairment, participation, environment, personal/emotional factors, and quality of life, as many of the interventions could have effects across domains. For example, research has demonstrated decreased language impairment after intervention targeting conversational participation in a group format (Elman & Bernstein-Ellis, 1999b).

The Comprehensive Aphasia Test (CAT; Swinburn, Porter, & Howard, 2004) and apraxia battery would be repeated to document changes in GJ's aphasia and apraxia of speech. In addition, functional-social approaches require demonstration of changes in "real life" performance, as opposed to changes in the *ability* to do something or to perform in restricted settings (e.g., clinic). Qualitative data collection will be repeated to describe outcomes in the categories of communicative behaviors, contexts, relationships, and subjective well-being (Simmons-Mackie & Damico, 1996, 2001a, 2001b). For example, the hypothetical contextual profile in Table–2 represents changes in participation after intervention. Similarly, a post-therapy social network diagram might demonstrate visible changes in the number, type and quality of social relationships in GJ's network (Figure 7–5). Videotapes of naturally occurring interactions (as described in assessment) are collected with the help of GJ's caregivers and family. In addition, videotapes of group therapy sessions, script enactments, conversations with trained partners, and other potential communicative situations are collected at the initiation of therapy, at intervals during therapy, and at the conclusion of a particular service to provide data for a range of discourse measures. For example, GJ's group participation can be judged over time in areas such as his number of conversational exchanges, variety and success of resources and strategies used (e.g., AAC, interactional strategies), number of topic initiations, number of content units communicated, inventory of speech acts used via any modality (e.g., questioning, commenting, greeting), or efficiency of repairs. In addition, videotape analysis can provide outcome data on changes in interactions with partners and changes in communicative environments. The participation questions of the AIA may also be repeated to determine change in participation and satisfaction regarding participation. Outcomes of intervention aimed at consequences of aphasia may also be measured by achievement of goals. GJ's achievement of participation goals may be tracked by personally relevant Goal Attainment Scales (Schlosser, 2004).. For example, Lasker, LaPointe, and Kodras (2005) report on the outcome of therapy to aid a university professor with aphasia in returning to teaching. The fact that the professor did, in fact, return to teaching and was positively rated by her students was ample evidence of a successful outcome.

Pre- and postintervention ratings with the AusTOMs provide a global impression of outcomes in the areas of language and speech. The VASES, Affect Balance Scale, BOSS CAPD, or Satisfaction with Life Scale might provide pre- and post-therapy ratings in the realm of well-being and subjective emotional factors. Also, a functional

Table 7–2. GJ's Major Activities Prior to the Onset of Aphasia, at the Initial Interview, and After Intervention

Preonset Activities	Postonset Activities	Postintervention Activities
Visiting family	Visiting daughter	Visiting daughter
		E-mailing son and family
Walking dog (Titch)		
		Keeping a journal
Reading newspaper	Reading newspaper	Reading newspaper
		Reading book and attending book club meetings
		Surfing the Internet
		E-mailing Internet "penpals"
Fishing		
Car repair		Car repair "advisor" to Aphasia group
Carpentry and home repair		
		Going to betting shop
Going to horse races and betting	Going to betting shop	Going to horse races with friend (volunteer partner)
Visiting the pub		Visiting the pub
		Aphasia speaker's bureau meetings

assessment consisting of the ASHA FACS would provide data on changes in performance of functional daily activities.

Of note, regarding outcome measurement is the philosophical issue of what is a "successful" outcome (Morris, Howard, & Kennedy, 2004). Functional-social approaches place importance on the

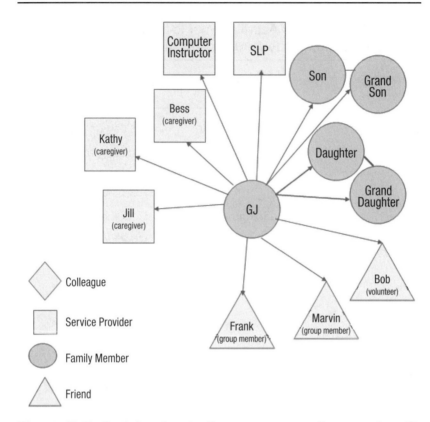

Figure 7–5. Social network diagram representing people with whom GJ regularly interacts after functional-social intervention (from CPS, Simmons-Mackie & Damico, 2001a).

client's subjective impressions of outcome as much as the clinician's objective measurement of outcome. Therefore, outcome measures include client perspectives, clinician judgments, and formal tests to document change.

Summary

This chapter has outlined hypothetical assessment and intervention for a person with severe apraxia of speech and aphasia. The intervention reflects a philosophical orientation and values consistent with a functional-social approach to aphasia. Functional-social approaches to aphasia are designed to reduce communication disability, promote life participation, and foster personal well-being. In defining social approaches to aphasia, Simmons-Mackie (2000, 2001a) notes that intervention is not necessarily directed only at social activities; rather functional-social approaches view aphasia within a sociocultural context. Because of the social significance of communication, disrupted communication entails social and psychological meanings and consequences. Functional-social approaches focus on the person with aphasia, people associated with the person with aphasia, the environment, and society at large. No single task or activity constitutes a functional-social approach. Intervention is determined by the values and beliefs of therapists as much as by the actual "activities" carried out in therapy (Byng & Duchan, 2005). For example, the belief that therapy should be client-centered and collaborative is a strong component of a social approach. The therapist and client act as partners in the therapy process with an emphasis on arriving at various "life goals" in the most effective, efficient, and pragmatic manner. A functional-social approach to therapy requires more than a clinic room and a knowledgeable therapist. It requires developing a network of people, organizations, or resources to support a wide-based intervention that will effect meaningful changes in the client's life.

References

Andersson, S., & Fridlund, B. (2002). The aphasic person's views of the encounter with other poeple: A grounded theory analysis. *Journal of Psychiatric and Mental Health Nursing, 9*, 285–292.

Astrom, M., Asplund, K., & Astrom, T. (1992). Psychosocial function and life satisfaction after stroke. *Stroke, 23*(4), 527–531.

Avent, J., & Austermann, S. (2003). Reciprocal scaffolding: A context for communication treatment in aphasia. *Aphasiology, 17*(4), 397–404.

Bellaire, K. Georges, J., & Thompson, C. (1991). Establishing functional communication board use for nonverbal aphasic subjects. *Clinical Aphasiology, 19*, 219–227.

Bernstein-Ellis, E., & Elman, R. (2006). *The Book Connection™: A life participation book club for individuals with acquired reading impairment, Manual.* Oakland, CA: Aphasia Center of California. Available at www.aphasiacenter.org

Bernstein-Ellis, E., & Elman, R. (2007). Aphasia Communication Group Treatment: The Aphasia Center of California Approach. In R. Elman

(Ed.), *Group treatment of neurogenic communication disorders: The expert clinician's approach* (2nd ed., pp. 71–94). San Diego, CA: Plural Publishing.

Boles, L. (1997). Conversation analysis as a dependent measure in communication therapy with aphasia. *Asia Pacific Journal of Speech, Language, and Hearing, 2,* 43–61.

Boles, L. (1998). Conversational discourse analysis as a method for evaluating progress in aphasia: A case report. *Journal of Communication Disorders, 31,* 261–274.

Booth, S., & Perkins, L. (1999). The use of conversation analysis to guide individualized advice to carers and evaluate change in aphasia: A case study. *Aphasiology, 13*(4–5), 283–303.

Bradburn, N. (1969). *The structure of psychological well-being.* Chicago: Aldine.

Brumfitt, S. (1993). Losing your sense of self: what aphasia can do. *Aphasiology, 7*(6), 569–575.

Brumfitt, S., & Sheeran, P. (1999). *The visual assessment of self-esteem scale.* Bicester, Oxford: Winslow Press.

Byng, S., & Duchan, J. (2005). Social model philosophies and principles: Their applications to therapies for aphasia. *Aphasiology, 19*(10–11), 906–922.

Byng, S., Pound, C., & Parr, S. (2000). Living with aphasia: A framework for therapy interventions. In I. Papathanasiou (Ed.), *Acquired neurological communication disorders: A clinical perspective* (pp. 49–75). London: Whurr.

Cranfill, T., Simmons-Mackie, N., & Kearns, K. (2005). Preface to "Treatment of aphasia through family member training." *Aphasiology, 19*(6), 577–581.

Cruice, M., Worrall, L., Hickson, L., & Murison, R. (2003). Finding a focus for quality of life in aphasia: Social and emotional health, and psychological well-being. *Aphasiology, 17*(4), 333–354.

Cruice, M., Worrall, L., Hickson, L., & Murison, R. (2005). Measuring quality of life: Comparing family members' and friends' ratings with those of their aphasic partners. *Aphasiology, 19*(2), 111–129.

Davidson, B., Worrall, L., & Hickson, L. (2006). Social communication in older age: Lessons from people with aphasia. *Topics in Stroke Rehabilitation, 13,* 1–13.

Diener, E., Emmons, R., Larsen, J., & Griffin, S. (1985). The Satisfaction with Life Scale. *Journal of Personality Assessment, 49*(1), 71–75.

Doyle, P. (2005). Advancing the development and understanding of patient-based outcomes in persons with aphasia. *Neurophysiology and Neurogenic Speech and Language Disorders, (ASHA Division 2), 15*(4), 7–9.

Doyle, P., McNeil, M. Hula, W., & Mikolic, J (2003) The Burden of Stroke Scale (BOSS): Validating patient-reported communication difficulty and associated psychological distress in stroke survivors, *Aphasiology, 17*, 291–304.

Duchan, J. F. (2001). Impairment and social views of speech-language pathology: Clinical practice re-examined. *Advances in Speech-Language Pathology, 3*(1), 37–46.

Duchan, J., & Black, M. (2001). Progressing toward life goals: A person-centered approach to evaluating therapy. *Topics in Language Disorders, 22*(1), 37–49.

Eadie, T., Yorkston, K., Klasner, E., Dudgeon, B., Deitz, J., Baylor, C., et al. (2006). Measuring communicative participation: A review of self-report instruments in speech-language pathology. *American Journal of Speech-Language Pathology, 15*(4), 307–320.

Elman, R. J. (2005). Social and life participation approaches to aphasia intervention In L. LaPointe (Ed.), *Aphasia and related neurogenic communication disorders* (3rd. ed.). New York: Thieme.

Elman, R., & Bernstein-Ellis, E. (1999a). Psychosocial aspects of group communication treatment. *Seminars in Speech and Language, 20*, 65–72.

Elman, R. J., & Bernstein-Ellis, E. (1999b). The efficacy of group communication treatment in adults with chronic aphasia. *Journal of Speech, Language, and Hearing Research, 42*, 411–419.

Finkelstein, V. (1991). Disability: An administrative challenge. In M. Oliver (Ed.), *Social work, disabled people and disabling environments* (pp. 19–39). London: Jessica Kinglsey.

Fougeyrollas, P., Noreau, L., Bergeron, H., Cloutier, R., Dion, S., & St-Michel, G. (1998). Social consequences of long term impairments and disabilities: Conceptual approach and assessment of handicap. *International Journal of Rehabilitation Research, 21*(2), 127–141.

Frattali, C., Thompson, C., Holland, A., Wohl, C., & Ferketic, M. (1995). *The American Speech-Language-Hearing Association Functional Assessment of Communication Skills for Adults (ASHA FACS)*. Rockville, MD: American Speech-Language-Hearing Association.

Garrett, K., & Beukelman, D. (1995). Changes in the interaction patterns of an individual with sever aphasia given three types of partner support. In R. Brookshire (Ed.), *Clinical aphasiology* (Vol. 23, pp. 237–251). Minneapolis, MN: BRK.

Garrett, K., & Beukelman, D. (1998). Adults with severe aphasia. In D. Beukelman, & P. Mirenda (Eds.), *Augmentative and alternative communication: management of severe communication disorders in children and adults* (2nd ed., pp. 465–500). Baltimore: Paul Brookes Publishing.

Goodwin, C. (1995). Co-constructing meaning in conversations with an aphasic man. *Research on Language and Social Interaction, 28,* 233–260.

Hafsteinsdottir, T. B., & Grypdonck, M. (1997). Being a stroke patient: A review of the literature. *Journal of Advanced Nursing, 26,* 580–588.

Haley, K., Jenkins, K., Hadden, C., Womack, J., Hall, J., & Schweiker, C. (2005). Sorting pictures to assess participation in life activities. *Neurophysiology and Neurogenic Speech and Language Disorders: ASHA Special Interest Division 2, 15*(4), 11–15.

Herrmann, M., & Wallesch, C.-W. (1989). Psychosocial changes and psychosocial adjustment with chronic and severe non-fluent aphasia. *Aphasiology, 3*(6), 513–526.

Hickey, E., Bourgeois, M., & Olswang, L. (2004). Effects of training volunteers to converse with nursing home residents with aphasia. *Aphasiology, 18*(5/6/7), 625–637.

Hinckley, J., & Packard, M. (2001). Family education seminars and social functioning in adults with chronic aphasia. *Journal of Communication Disorders, 34,* 241–254.

Ho, K., Weiss, S., Garrett, K., & Lloyd, L. (2005). The effect of remnant and pictographic books on the communicative interaction of individuals with global aphasia. *Augmentative and Alternative Communication, 21*(3), 218–232.

Holland, A. (1982) Observing functional communication of aphasic adults, *Journal of Speech and Hearing Disorders, 47,* 50–56.

Hopper, T., & Holland, A. (1998). Situation-specific training for adults with aphasia: An example. *Aphasiology, 12,* 933–944.

Hopper, T., Holland, A., & Rewega, M. (2002). Conversational coaching: treatment outcomes and future directions. *Aphasiology, 16,* 745–762.

Kagan, A., Black, S., Duchan, J., Simmons-Mackie, N., & Square, P. (2001). Training volunteers as conversation partners using "supported conversation for adults with aphasia" (SCA): A controlled trial. *Journal of Speech, Language and Hearing Research, 44*(3), 624–638.

Kagan, A., & Gailey, G. (1993). Functional is not enough: Training conversation partners in aphasia. In A. Holland & M. Forbes (Eds.), *Aphasia treatment: World perspectives* (pp. 199–226). San Diego, CA: Singular Publishing Group.

Kagan, A., Simmons-Mackie, N., Rowland, A., Huijbregts, M., Shumway E., McEwen, S., et al. (in press). Counting what counts: A framework for capturing real-life outcomes of aphasia intervention. *Aphasiology.*

Kagan, A., Simmons-Mackie, N., Rowland, A., Huijbregts, M., Shumway E., McEwen, S., et al. (unpublished). *Aphasia Institute Assessment.*

Kagan, A., Winckel, J., & Shumway, E. (1996). *Pictographic communication resources.* North York, Canada: Pat Arato Aphasia Centre.

Kovarsky, D., Kimbarow, M., & Kastner, D. (1999). Group language therapy practice among adults with traumatic brain injury. In D. Kovarsky, J. Duchan, & M. Maxwell (Eds.), *Constructing (In) competence: Disabling evaluations in clinical and social interaction* (pp. 291-312). Hillsdale, NJ: Lawrence Erlbaum.

Lasker, J., LaPointe, L., & Kodras, J. (2005). Helping a professor with aphasia resume teaching through multimodal approaches. *Aphasiology, 19*(3-5), 399-410.

Lock, S., Wilkinson, R., Bryan, K., Maxim, J., Edmundson, A., & Bruce, C. (2001). Supporting partners of people with aphasia in relationships and conversation (SPPARC). *International Journal of Language and Communication Disorders, 36*, 25-30.

Lomas, J., Pickard, L., & Mohide, A. (1987). Patient versus clinician item generation for quality-of-life measures. *Medical Care, 25*(8), 764-769.

LPAA Project Group (in alphabetical order Chapey, R., Duchan, J. F., Elman, R. J., Garcia, L. J., Kagan, A., Lyon, J., & Simmons-Mackie, N. (2000). Life participation approach to aphasia: Looking to the future. *ASHA Leader, 5*(3), 4-6.

LPAA Project Group. (2001). Life participation approach to aphasia: A statement of values for the future. In R. Chapey (Ed.), *Language intervention strategies in aphasia and related neurogenic communication disorders* (4th ed., pp. 235-245). Philadelphia: Lippincott, Williams & Wilkins.

Lubinski, R. (2001). Environmental systems approach to adult aphasia . In R. Chapey (Ed.), *Language intervention strategies in aphasia and related neurogenic communication disorders* (pp. 269-296). Philadelphia: Lippincott, Williams & Wilkins.

Lyon, J. (1996). Optimizing communication and participation in life for aphasic adults and their prime caregivers in natural settings: A use model for treatment. In G. Wallace (Ed.), *Adult aphasia rehabilitation* (pp. 137-160). Newton, MA: Butterworth-Heinemann.

Lyon, J. G., Carisk, D., Keisler, L., Rosenbek, J., Levine, R., Kumpula, J., et al. (1997). Communication partners: Enhancing participation in life and communication for adults with aphasia in natural settings. *Aphasiology, 11*, 693-708.

Morris, J., Howard, D., & Kennedy, S. (2004). The value of therapy: What counts? In J. Duchan & S. Byng (Eds.), *Challenging aphasia therapies* (pp. 134-157). New York: Psychology Press.

Morris, M., Perry, A., Unsworth, C., Skeat, J., Taylor, N., Dodd, K., et al. (2005). Reliability of the Australian Therapy Outcome Measures for quantifying outcomes in disability and health. *International Journal of Therapy and Rehabilitation, 12*, 340-346.

Muller, D. (1999). Managing psychosocial adjustment to aphasia. *Seminars in Speech and Language, 20*, 85-92.

National Joint Committee for the Communication Needs of Persons with Severe Disabilities (NJC). (1992). Guidelines for meeting the communication needs of persons with severe disabilities. *Asha, 34* (Suppl. 7), 2-3.

Oelschlaeger, M., & Damico, J. S. (2000). Partnership in conversation: A study of word search strategies. *Journal of Communication Disorders, 33*, 205-225.

Oliver, M. (1996). *Understanding disability: From theory to practice.* London: Macmillan.

Parr, S., & Byng, S. (2000). Perspectives and priorities: Accessing user views in functional communication assessment. In L. Worrall & C. Frattali (Eds.), *Neurogenic communication disorders: A functional approach* (pp. 55-66). New York: Thieme.

Perry, A., Morris, M., Unsworth, C., Duckett, S., Skeat, J., Dodd, K., et al. (2004). Therapy outcome measures for allied health practitioners in Australia: The AusTOMs. *International Journal for Quality in Health Care, 16*, 285-291.

Pound, C., Parr, S., Lindsay, J., & Woolf, C. (2000). *Beyond aphasia: Therapies for living with communication disability.* Bicester, UK: Speechmark.

Purdy, M., & Hindenlang, J. (2005). Educating and training caregivers of persons with aphasia. *Aphasiology, 19*, 377-388.

Rayner, H., & Marshall, J. (2003). Training volunteers as conversation partners for people with aphasia. *International Journal of Language and Communication Disorders, 38*, 149-164.

Rogers, M. (2001). Treatment research on augmentative and alternative communication for adults with apraxia of speech. *Neurophysiology and Neurogenic Speech and Language Disorders, ASHA SID 2, 11*(4), 21-27.

Ross, K., & Wertz, T. (2003). Quality of life with and without aphasia. *Aphasiology, 17*, 335-364.

Sarno, M. T. (2004). Aphasia therapies: Historical perspectives and moral imperatives. In J. Duchan & S. Byng (Eds.), *Challenging aphasia therapies* (pp. 17-31). Hove, UK: Psychology Press.

Schlosser, R. (2004). Goal attainment scaling as a clinical measurement technique in communication disorders: A critical review. *Journal of Communication Disorders, 37*, 217-239.

Shadden, B. (2005). Aphasia as identity theft: Theory and practice. *Aphasiology, 19*, 211-223.

Simmons-Mackie, N. (1988). A trip down Easy Street. *Clinical Aphasiology, 18*, 19-30.

Simmons-Mackie, N. (1998a). A solution to the discharge dilemma in aphasia: Social approaches to aphasia management. *Aphasiology, 12*, 231–239.

Simmons-Mackie, N. (1998b). In support of supported communication for adults with aphasia: Clinical forum. *Aphasiology, 12*, 831–838.

Simmons-Mackie, N. (2000). Social approaches to the management of aphasia. In L. Worrall & C. Frattali (Eds.), *Neurogenic communication disorders: A functional approach* (pp. 162–187). New York, Thieme.

Simmons-Mackie, N. (2001a). Social approaches to aphasia intervention. In R. Chapey (Ed), *Language intervention strategies in aphasia and related neurogenic communication disorders* (4th ed., pp. 246–268). Philadelphia: Lippincott, Williams & Wilkins.

Simmons-Mackie, N. (2001b). Social approaches to clinical practice: Examining clinical assumptions. *Advances in Speech-Language Pathology, 3*(1), 47–50.

Simmons-Mackie, N. (2004). Just kidding! Humour and therapy for aphasia. In J. Duchan & S. Byng (Eds.), *Challenging aphasia therapies* (pp. 101–117). New York: Psychology Press.

Simmons-Mackie, N., & Damico, J. (1995). Communicative competence in aphasia: Evidence from compensatory strategies. *Clinical Aphasiology, 23*, 95–105.

Simmons-Mackie, N., & Damico, J. (1996a). Accounting for handicaps in aphasia: Communicative assessment from an authentic social perspective. *Disability and Rehabilitation, 18*, 540–549.

Simmons-Mackie, N., & Damico, J. (1996b). The contribution of discourse markers to communicative competence in aphasia. *American Journal of Speech-Language Pathology, 5*, 37–43.

Simmons-Mackie, N., & Damico, J. S. (2001a). *Communicative profiling system: Descriptive assessment of social interaction in aphasia.* Workshop presented at the British Aphasiology Society Meeting.

Simmons-Mackie, N., & Damico, J. S. (2001b). Intervention outcomes: Clinical application of qualitative methods. *Topics in Language Disorders, 21*, 21–36.

Simmons-Mackie, N., Elman, R., Holland, A., & Damico, J. (2007). Management of discourse in group therapy for aphasia. *Topics in Language Disorders, 27*, 5–23.

Simmons-Mackie, N., & Kagan, A. (1999). Communication strategies used by "good" versus "poor" speaking partners of individuals with aphasia. *Aphasiology, 13*, 807–820.

Simmons-Mackie, N., Kearns, K., & Potechin, G. (2005/1987). CAC Classics: Treatment of aphasia through family member training. *Aphasiology, 19*(6), 583–593.

Simmons-Mackie, N., Kingston, D., & Schultz, M. (2005). "Speaking for another": The management of participation frames in aphasia. *American Journal of Speech-Language Pathology, 13*, 114–127.

Sorin-Peters, R. (2004). The evaluation of learner-centered training programme for spouses of adults with aphasia. *Aphasiology, 18*(10), 951–975.

Spradley, J. P. (1979). *The ethnographic interview.* New York: Holt, Rinehart and Winston.

Swinburn, K., Porter, G., & Howard, D. (2004). *Comprehensive Aphasia Test.* New York: Psychology Press.

Unsworth, C., Duckett, S., Duncombe, D., Perry, A., Skeat, J., & Taylor, N. (2004). Validity of the AusTOM Scales: A comparison of the AusTOMs and EuroQol-5D. *Health and Quality of Life Outcomes, 2*(1), 64.

Wambaugh, J. (2001). Sound production treatment for Apraxia of Speech. *Neurophysiology and Neurogenic Speech and Language Disorders, ASHA SID 2,* 11(4), 9–13.

Westby, C. E. (1990). Ethnographic interviewing: Asking the right questions to the right people in the right ways. *Journal of Childhood Communication Disorders, 13*(1), 101–111.

Westby, C., Burda, A., & Mehta, Z. (2003). Asking the right questions in the right ways. *ASHA Leader, 8*(8), 4–5; 16–17.

World Health Organization (WHO). (2001). *International Classification of Functioning, Disability and Health (ICF).* Geneva, Switzerland.

Worrall, L. (2000). A conceptual framework for a functional approach to acquired neurogenic disorders of communication and swallowing. In L. Worrall & C. Frattali (Eds.), *Neurogenic communication disorders: A functional approach* (pp. 3–18). New York: Thieme.

Worrall, L., Rose, T., Howe, T., McKenna, K., & Hickson, L. (2007). Developing an evidence-base for accessibility for people with aphasia. *Aphasiology, 21*(1), 124–136.

Youmans, G., Holland, A., Munoz, M., & Bourgeois, M. (2005). Script training and automaticity in two individuals with aphasia. *Aphasiology, 19*(3–5), 435–450.

8

Treatment for a Case of Severe Apraxia of Speech and Aphasia

An Impairment-Based Perspective

David Howard

Introduction

GJ has considerable strengths: although his voluntary production of language is extremely limited, testing with the New England Panto-mime Test (Duffy & Duffy, 1984) shows that he has both good comprehension and production of gesture. His language comprehension is also good: his single word comprehension is within normal limits, with both spoken and written words, although he is mildly impaired in spoken sentence comprehension.

In this chapter, I discuss how a speech language pathologist might approach treatment. First, some considerations about the content and targets of therapy, and then some consideration on how it might be delivered are discussed, thinking particularly about "service delivery" at the Newcastle Aphasia Centre in Newcastle, England.

It has to be taken as central that, whatever one's perspective, the aims of aphasia therapy are (1) to facilitate the most effective communication possible, whatever the means, and (2) to work with the client to maximize their ability to participate in social interactions, at any level. Howard and Hatfield (1987) argue that the problem for "social" approaches to aphasia therapy is that they confuse means and ends. The question that divides "social" and "impairment-based" approaches to aphasia therapy is not about aims, but about means. At its most extreme position an exponent of the social approach might argue that therapy always has to be based in real-life communication. The impairment-based position might be quite different: although the *aim* will be better communication, the *means* of achieving this would be development of the component skills.

It is clear that one has to distinguish aims and means. Consider an example: in learning a musical instrument, a student spends a great deal of time in learning scales. This is not because scales improve the production of music directly or that the long-term aim is being able to produce scales, but because producing them develops skills (in this case motor patterns) that are important for real music production. In short, we know that component skills can be learned divorced from their functional outcome.

In what follows, then, I take as axiomatic that the aims of aphasia therapy cannot be identified with the means; all approaches seek to provide the client with the means to improve their communication. I also take as axiomatic that aphasia therapy should be motivated by knowledge of both strengths and weaknesses (intact and impaired processes); these strengths and weaknesses can be described both in terms of communication, and in terms of language processing. To seek their sources we have to consider the underlying impairments.

The point of doing so is not that, from any perspective, knowledge of a client's language processing strengths and weaknesses and identification of their underlying impairments, can *determine* the best therapy. As Basso and Marangolo (2000) put it:

> The most important contribution of cognitive neuropsychology to aphasia therapy lies in the massive reduction of the theoretically-motivated choices left open to the therapist. Clearly articulated and detailed hypotheses about representations and processing of cognitive functions allow rejection of all those strategies for treatment that are not theoretically justified. The more detailed the cognitive model, the narrower the spectrum of rationally motivated treat-

ments; whereas the less fine-grained the cognitive model, the greater the number of theoretically justifiable therapeutic interventions
(p. 203).

So, what good assessment does is reduce the space of choice of therapy methods.

The choice of approach should also be evidence-based; that is,
one should be guided in choosing treatment approaches by the results of the best available treatment studies involving patients with
qualitatively similar disorders, and addressed toward the same underlying impairment(s). And these treatment studies need to be
able to deliver impacts with the same aims as sought with an individual client.

The problem here is that there is little, if any, relevant evidence
from existing treatment studies, for people with severe aphasia.
This is not an unusual position in therapy with people with neuropsychological disorders, but it is uncomfortable. By default, one
is forced to choose treatment methods on the basis of their logical
form, their fit with neuropsychological theory, and their intended
benefits without any real confidence, from existing empirical studies, that they will prove to be effective.

Central to any approach to treatment is negotiation of the *aims*
of treatment. What does the client seek to achieve through aphasia therapy and how does this relate to what the therapist thinks
that she or he can deliver? The subtlety of this negotiation should
not be underestimated. GJ may, for example, want to achieve normal language production, but this is unrealistic. Almost all people
with a 4-year history of severe aphasia will continue to have substantial language impairments. A more realistic aim, perhaps, is to
seek to improve the linguistic resources that he can use in communication with the aim of making it as effective and satisfying as possible (Peach, 2001).

Case Interpretation and Additional
Assessment to Identify the Underlying Deficit

On testing, GJ has normal or close to normal comprehension of
both spoken and written language, and functionally he feels he has
no difficulty. There is no obvious justification for further investiga-
tion of comprehension. It is possible that he does have some diffi-

culty with reversible sentences presented in a test format, but given that such sentences in context are usually unambiguously interpretable this is unlikely to have any impact.

GJ has little spoken output. Is this a problem that can be localized to articulatory programming—that is, a "purely apraxic" disorder? Or is there also a more central difficulty in word retrieval? It is necessary to investigate whether he has access to a phonological specification of a word, even when he cannot produce it in spoken form. The obvious way of doing this is using a task that requires access to phonology without spoken output. Candidate assessments are picture homophone judgments (e.g., judging that a picture of a "stake" and a "steak" sound the same) or homophone judgments with written words (easier to generate satisfactory stimuli; e.g., judging that *so* and *sew* are homophones but that *no* and *new* are not) (see Coltheart, Masterson, Byng, Prior, & Riddoch, 1983; Nickels, Howard, & Best, 1997; Whitworth, Webster, & Howard, 2005 for discussion). Good performance in these tasks would show that GJ can access lexical phonological representations for words, and that his problem is postlexical (plausibly in generating an articulatory motor program). Poor performance would suggest that his problem in generating spoken production is not only at a postlexical level.

This is important for two reasons: first, if spoken production is targeted in therapy, an approach where articulatory production only is targeted may be less successful if his difficulties are both lexical and articulatory. Second, good access to phonological representations will have impact on how one might address therapy for writing.

In comparison to spoken language production, GJ's writing is a strength. He is accurate in written naming of around 50% of pictures (although he is worse with longer words), and can, with some difficulty, write messages. But this raises the question of how he generates written words. Is this lexical writing? That is, is it based on lexical orthographic representations retrieved directly from semantics? Or is he generating an (internal) phonological specification and using this to drive his written responses?

Distinguishing these possibilities will have implications for intervention. If GJ's writing is based on internally generated phonology, a sensible therapy strategy would be to try to improve phonological-to-orthographic conversion mechanisms. An advantage of this is that any improvement would be expected to generalize, as phonological-to-orthographic conversion mechanisms can be applied to any phonological string. If his writing is purely lexically driven, any therapy directed to improving spelling would have only item-specific effects (because the semantics-to-orthography relationship is arbitrary: knowing that $cat_{semantics}$ is spelled *C-A-T* does not help with knowing that $dog_{semantics}$ is spelled *D-O-G*). If that is the case, and therapy effects are likely to be item-specific, any attempt to improve his writing would be best directed toward words that are likely to be functionally useful.

How to do this? Writing nonwords to dictation would test his ability to convert sublexically between phonology and orthography. Writing homophones to dictation with a disambiguating context (e.g., "Write berry; a berry is a fruit") would be revealing. If he makes homophone errors (e.g., writing *bury*) it would show that his writing is mediated by lexical phonological representations. Errors in writing to dictation would also be informative. If GJ makes phonologically plausible errors (e.g. writing *spear* as *speer* or *spere*) it would support phonological mediation.

And why is GJ more accurate in writing short words than long words? There are two possibilities; the first is that long words are simply more vulnerable. Because they have more letters a corruption of lexical orthographic representations would necessarily result in poorer accuracy with longer words. There is another possibility, though. Writing takes time, and so the orthographic specification has to be maintained in the graphemic output buffer. If there is a deficit at this level, there will be decay of the representation. This should result in poorer performance with longer words.

How can these possibilities be distinguished? Nonwords have no lexical representation, so they should be affected only by impairment to the graphemic output buffer. So if there is an equal length effect with words and nonwords in writing to dictation, there is evidence in favor of impairment at a level shared by words and nonwords—the graphemic output buffer. If the length effect is more marked with real words than nonwords, it is likely that the effect is due to corruption of lexical orthographic representations.

So, it is necessary to investigate GJ's writing in more detail. This is because the results will give information about the level at which he has difficulty, which, in turn, will determine what are sensible therapy approaches.

Considering writing, we need to know how he copes with more complex tasks than picture naming. When a sentence is needed, how does he do? Does he omit function words or produce them correctly? This is important because it impacts on his ability to use writing effectively in communication.

There is no information on GJ's drawing abilities. It would be important to assess this as drawing can be an important source of effective information in communication.

Treatment

As a result of his aphasia, GJ has very severe communication problems. But, in real life, there are many things that he can do well. He has good comprehension of both spoken and written language; he watches television, reads the newspaper, and places bets on the horses with pleasure.

His limiting difficulties are with language production: he can say reliably only "aye" and "no." Yet he has considerable resources; he can produce gesture accurately. He can write many words accurately. And his comprehension of spoken and written language is (more-or-less) unimpaired.

Thinking about outcomes, any sensible aim would be to optimize his language output from speech, writing, gesture, and drawing, and to recruit all of his resources toward successful communication. There are a number of themes that should be addressed in therapy, related to spoken output, written output, and the use of alternative augmentative communication (AAC) systems. These are discussed below.

Spoken Output

GJ's ability to produce speech is severely limited, although the little that he uses consistently is communicatively effective. Although he is 4 years postonset, it is worth trying to improve his spoken output. We have seen substantial improvements in spoken output when systematic work on articulatory production was initiated as many as 7 years postonset, although the most frequent outcome in people with chronic aphasia is little improvement. In communicative terms, spoken production is the most useful form of output, and so any progress in this domain will be beneficial.

The evidence on therapy effectiveness for profound apraxia is both equivocal and limited (see Duffy, 2005 for review). Crudely, there are two primary alternatives for treatment of apraxia of speech; these are synthetic and holistic approaches.

A Synthetic Approach

This works from simple articulatory gestures (individual phonemes) and aims to build these up into syllables, then words, then phrases. Early work can be shaped using articulograms, illustrating the target articulatory positions for individual phonemes (Varley & Whiteside, 2001). It might also use GJ's relatively intact ability to produce articulatory gestures in nonspeech movements to shape similar speech productions (e.g., a blowing out candles movement can be used to elicit a /p/ production).

The Holistic Approach

This approach contrasts with the synthetic approach by aiming for production of whole phrases (or words or syllables) aiming more for recognizable production than segmental accuracy. The targets used should obviously be chosen in terms of their utility in communication: were GJ to improve here and if his improvement were item specific, communicatively effective targets would, obviously, be most useful.

Both of these approaches should, probably, be used in conjunction. There seems to be no published evidence that either is more effective than the other, or indeed that either is likely to be effective in severe speech apraxia. In this case it seems sensible to put one's eggs in both baskets. Any improvement as a result of either approach could be of real benefit to the client.

Although improvement in spoken output is likely to be most effective in terms of improving GJ's ability to communicate (and thus worth the effort), substantial change is, both on the basis of the literature and our experience, unlikely though not impossible. Therapy, therefore, needs also to address other means of communication.

Written Output

GJ has some writing ability: he can write the names of a substantial variety of pictures and when he makes errors they are likely to be target related and so communicatively effective. .An obvious target in therapy is to improve his writing ability, especially for words that are likely to be of use in communication. As indicated above, the approach to this problem should be constrained by the nature of his writing difficulties. If GJ is primarily generating written responses on the basis of internal phonology, when his access to phonological representations is relatively intact, this would generate phonologically plausible, although orthographically incorrect, responses (e.g., *train* → *trane*); these would, however, be both informative and incorrect. If writing were to depend on phonology, therapy could concentrate on developing phonological-to-orthographic conversion (both phoneme-to-letter rules and rules relating phonemes to graphemes—groups of letters, e.g., /tʃ/ → ch) (Hillis & Caramazza, 1994; Luzzatti, Colombo, Frustaci, & Vitolo, 2000). In this case, where writing is mediated by relatively intact access to phonological representations, working on phoneme-to-grapheme relationships would deliver improvements that are item independent. That is, the results should generalize to any item containing the treated correspondences.

If writing is lexically driven, therapy would be sensibly concentrated on improving these lexically driven responses. In this case, any improvement is likely to be lexically specific—that is, resulting in improvement only in treated words. There is, therefore, an imperative to target words that are likely to be functionally useful. Appropriate methods are likely to include: copy and recall (CART therapy), anagrams and recall, or possibly the use of visual imagery strategies (Beeson, 1999; Beeson, Hirsch, & Rewega, 2002; De Partz, Seron, & Van der Linden, 1992; Rapp & Beeson, 2003; Rapp & Kane, 2002). Given that GJ's comprehension of written words is good, there is the possibility of developing a personalized writing dictionary. GJ would have a book containing words that he is likely to want to use, organized in a way that he finds useful (perhaps by initial letter, or by category, or by both). As van de Sandt-Koenderman (2004) emphasizes, "for a personalised vocabulary it is necessary that it is continuously updated to reflect current needs. In this process of vocabulary selection, the therapist should work together with the client and their family and friends, interviewing them about communicative needs" (Worrall, 1999)" (p. 251).

Alternative and Augmentative Communication

GJ has been provided with a sophisticated communication device that can produce spoken words and sentences when a key is pressed, but he is reluctant to use it. An issue to investigate is why he does not use it. Is it because he cannot (he does not understand—perhaps because of language processing difficulties—how to use it) or because he is dissatisfied with the nature of the communication it provides?

Many people with aphasia are reluctant to use alternative communication devices because they are not real speech (van de Sandt-Koenderman, 2004). Nevertheless, for those capable of using them, they give the opportunity to produce appropriate sentences. The difficulty is that it may be difficult in real time to respond to the response from another. That is, while one can generate a sentence/utterance off-line in anticipation of an interaction, it may be much harder to engage in a real interaction.

So how is one to develop GJ's ability to engage in real communicative interactions? The answer lies in "total communication" (Lawson & Fawcus, 1999). That is, developing his ability to use *all* of his communicative resources in the service of effective communication. Consider his resources: First, he can gesture well; second, he can write with some accuracy the names of many targets. There is no information about his drawing abilities, but it is possible to consider whether his drawing abilities can be used in communication (Hatfield & Zangwill, 1974; Lyon, 1995; Sacchett, Byng, Marshall, & Pound, 1999). He has good written word comprehension, so he should be able to use a personalized communication book to choose appropriate words to convey his message. Finally, GJ can verbally indicate "yes" and "no" accurately verbally.

The aim of therapy would be for GJ to use all his resources in the service of communication. One way of approaching this would be using the methods described by Davis and Wilcox in PACE (Promoting Aphasics' Communicative Effectiveness; (Davis, 1980; Davis

& Wilcox, 1981, 1985). This gives a framework for therapy where the therapist and the person with aphasia alternate in communicating messages that are unknown to the other. The therapist can use his or her turn to model possible communicative strategies, and, can give the person with aphasia real feedback on the effectiveness of their responses. An advantage of this approach is that the therapist can, by choosing appropriate therapy materials, vary the complexity of the message that needs to be conveyed.

In addition, treatment could initially focus on individual aspects of communication (i.e., drawing, writing, gesture, verbal yes/no responses, a communication book/dictionary) and then move toward bringing them together (i.e., using them in conjunction), and developing flexibility in choosing the most appropriate method to use depending on the topic and resources (Yoshihata, Watamori, Chujo, & Masuyama, 1998). The long-term aim would be to use all of these resources effectively in real time in the service of communication. Individually, each of these methods is likely to be inadequate; as van de Sandt-Koenderman (2004) writes about gesture, "gestures are often ambiguous, and can only refer to a reduced set of—mainly concrete—concepts. Often the gestures are only comprehensible in the situational context. It is easy to use the gesture to ask for a hammer when standing next to a toolbox, but it is difficult to refer to the fact that you have been a biotechnologist or that you worry about your daughter's health" (p. 247). Using all of these resources together and flexibly, gives a much better chance of being able to address successfully more complex topics

In conjunction with this one would want to consider training of conversational partners, in particular his daughter, and possibly his caregivers (Kagan, 1998; Turner & Whitworth, 2006a, 2006b). Using total communication requires inventiveness and flexibility from all the participants, a willingness to engage, and knowledge of GJ's resources and how he uses them most effectively.

Delivery of Treatment

Given that there is substantial evidence that more intensive therapy is more effective (Albert, 2003; Basso, 2003; Bhogal, Teasell, & Speechley, 2003), it would be best to provide therapy intensively. At the Newcastle Aphasia Centre, established by a cooperation between therapists in the University and adult Speech and Language

Therapy Services in the North-East of England, we are able to offer therapy for 3 days per week with five individual one-to-one therapy sessions (totaling 3 hrs, 45 min) a week together with 9 hrs, 45 min of group therapy over 3 days each week. Clients come, initially, for a 12-week course. This therapy regimen demands a considerable commitment from the clients, in terms of both time and effort. The deal we offer is that we do our best to deliver improvements in their speech, language, and communication and the clients need to agree to commit to the enterprise: to attend regularly, and agree to work as hard as they can.

Individual therapy can be used to work on the individual skills as described above, and then bringing them together in structured one-to-one exercises. The idea, as emphasized by many aphasia therapists including Luria (1947) and Seron (1979), is that it is important to both develop skills and practice them enough so that they become more automatic and less attention-demanding.

The role of the group is more subtle and less easily defined. As Kearns and Elman (2001) point out, group therapy can have many functions that can be combined—that is, several may be met simultaneously in any session. Our groups are deliberately relatively sparse; that is they include in addition to perhaps eight people with aphasia, usually only one or two helpers (volunteers who are often people with aphasia) in addition to the therapist who is "running" the group. This is deliberate: a group where most of the participants are people with aphasia puts most of the communicative load on the clients. As a result, it requires them to use, in a real communicative context, but one that is both supportive and tolerant, the skills that they have learned in individual sessions.

It also provides the opportunity to interact with other people with aphasia. This is important for a number of reasons. First, because aphasia causes social isolation, a group puts people with aphasia into contact with other people with aphasia. The benefit of realizing that others are in the same situation should not be underestimated. Solidarity and friendship really matter. It gives the opportunity of learning from others about what one can do as a person with aphasia; for example, one can realize that fishing is a possible activity with a language impairment. The client can also learn from the other people with aphasia about effective communication strategies. Seeing others using these strategies successfully within a group can motivate the person with aphasia to develop similar skills.

In a wider context, groups can, through building solidarity and sharing interests between people with aphasia, lead to action on a wider scale. At the Newcastle Aphasia Centre this has led to the development of a charity, NETA—the North-East Trust for Aphasia—that campaigns for facilities and resources for people with aphasia raises money, and runs support and educational groups for people with aphasia and their carers.

Summary

Any plan for therapy with GJ needs to capitalize on his strengths and address his difficulties while being guided by goals negotiated with him that both he and the therapists own. The overall aim must be to maximize his communication ability, and to enable him to engage in satisfying and effective interactions that allow him to engage in the activities he wants to do.

That is an aspiration, and a worthy aspiration, but it needs to be tempered by a realization that GJ has a severe aphasia and is extremely unlikely to regain anything approaching normal language. A realistic aim is to achieve the best communication possible and to hone his abilities to deal effectively with the kinds of communication contexts he most often encounters—with his family, with his carers, and, for example, in the betting shop.

His therapy must be constructed on the basis of an understanding of the nature of his difficulties in terms of language processing (Whitworth et al., 2005). For example, as argued above, the way in which writing might be recruited to help in communication will be constrained by the nature of his underlying impairment; similarly, therapy for his speech production impairment will be different if his difficulty is purely in postlexical articulatory programming (articulatory apraxia) or if a difficulty in lexical retrieval also contributes. Therapy with the potential of being effective can only be designed if the nature of his underlying impairments is properly understood.

Although treatment from therapists, guided by a clear analysis of his processing deficits and intact abilities, has much to offer GJ, it is important to realize that he may be able to learn a great deal from other people with aphasia about how to live in the real world with language impairments; this is something that can only happen in a group with other people with aphasia.

References

Albert, M. (2003). Intensity of aphasia therapy: Impact on recovery. *Stroke, 34*(4), 992–993.

Basso, A. (2003). *Aphasia and its therapy.* Oxford, UK: Oxford University Press.

Basso, A., & Marangolo, P. (2000). Cognitive neuropsychological rehabilitation: The emperor's new clothes? *Neuropsychological Rehabilitation, 10*(3), 219–229.

Beeson, P. M. (1999). Treating acquired writing impairment: strengthening graphemic representations. *Aphasiology, 13*(9–11), 767–785.

Beeson, P. M., Hirsch, F. M., & Rewega, M. A. (2002). Successful single-word writing treatment: Experimental analyses of four cases. *Aphasiology, 16*(4–6), 473–491.

Bhogal, S., Teasell, R., & Speechley, M. (2003). Intensity of aphasia therapy, impact on recovery. *Stroke, 34*(4), 987–993.

Coltheart, M., Masterson, J., Byng, S., Prior, M., & Riddoch, M. J. (1983). Surface dyslexia. *Quarterly Journal of Experimental Psychology, 35A,* 469–496.

Davis, G. A. (1980). A critical look at PACE therapy. In R. Brookshire (Ed.), *Clinical Aphasiology Conference proceedings* (Vol. 1980). Minneapolis, MN: BRK.

Davis, G. A., & Wilcox, M. J. (1981). Incorporating parameters of natural conversation in aphasia treatment. In R. Chapey (Ed.), *Language intervention strategies in adult aphasia* (pp. 161–194). Baltimore: Williams.

Davis, G. A., & Wilcox, M. J. (1985). *Adult aphasia rehabilitation: Applied pragmatics.* Windsor, UK: NFER-Nelson.

De Partz, M., Seron, X., & Van der Linden, M. (1992). Re-education of a surface dysgraphia with a visual imagery strategy. *Cognitive Neuropsychology, 9,* 369–401.

Duffy, J. R. (2005). *Motor speech disorders* (2nd. ed.). St. Louis, MO: Elsevier.

Duffy, R. J., & Duffy, J. R. (1984). *New England Pantomime Tests.* Austin, TX: Pro-Ed.

Hatfield, F. M., & Zangwill, O. L. (1974). Ideation in aphasia: the picture-story method. *Neuropsychologia, 12*(3), 389–393.

Hillis, A. E., & Caramazza, A. (1994). Theories of lexical processing and rehabilitation of lexical deficits. In M. J. Riddoch & G. W. Humphreys (Eds.), *Cognitive neuropsychology and cognitive rehabilitation* (pp. 449–482). London: Lawrence Erlbaum Associates.

Howard, D., & Hatfield, F. M. (1987). *Aphasia therapy: Historical and contemporary issues.* London: Lawrence Erlbaum.

Kagan, A. (1998). Supported conversation for adults with aphasia: Methods and resources for training conversation partners. *Aphasiology, 12,* 816–830.

Kearns, K. P., & Elman, R. J. (2001). Group therapy for aphasia: Theoretical and practical considerations. In R. Chapey (Ed.), *Language intervention strategies in aphasia and related neurogenic communication disorders* (4th ed., pp. 316–337). Baltimore: Lippincott, Williams and Wilkins.

Lawson, R., & Fawcus, M. (1999). Increasing effective communication using a total communication approach. In S. Byng & K. Swinburn, & C. Pound (Eds.), *The aphasia therapy file* (pp. 61–73). Hove, UK: Psychology Press.

Luria, A. R. (1947). *Traumatic aphasia* (Trans. from the Russian by D. Bowden 1970). The Hague: Mouton.

Luzzatti, C., Colombo, C., Frustaci, M., & Vitolo, F. (2000). Rehabilitation of spelling along the sub-word-level routine. *Neuropsychological Rehabilitation, 10*(3), 249–278.

Lyon, J. (1995). Drawing: Its value as a communication aid for adults with aphasia. *Aphasiology, 9,* 33–95.

Nickels, L. A., Howard, D., & Best, W. (1997). Fractionating the articulatory loop: Dissociations and associations in phonological recoding in aphasia. *Brain and Language, 56*(2), 161–182.

Peach, R. K. (2001). Clinical intervention for global aphasia. In R. Chapey (Ed.), *Language intervention strategies in aphasia and related neurogenic communication disorders* (4th ed., pp. 487–512). Baltimore: Lippincott Williams and Wilkins.

Rapp, B., & Beeson, P. (2003). Dysgraphia: Cognitive processes, remediation, and neural substrates—Introduction. *Aphasiology, 17*(6-7), 531–534.

Rapp, B., & Kane, A. (2002). Remediation of deficits affecting different components of the spelling process. *Aphasiology, 16*(4-6), 439–454.

Sacchett, C., Byng, S., Marshall, J., & Pound, C. (1999). Drawing together: Evaluation of a therapy programme for severe aphasia. *International Journal of Language and Communication Disorders, 34*(3), 265–289.

Seron, X. (1979). *Aphasie et neuropsychologie: Approches therapeutiques.* Brussels, Belgium: Mardaga.

Turner, S., & Whitworth, A. (2006a). Clinicians' perceptions of candidacy for conversation partner training in aphasia: How do we select candidates for therapy and do we get it right? *Aphasiology, 20*(7), 616–643.

Turner, S., & Whitworth, A. (2006b). Conversational partner training programmes in aphasia: A review of key themes and participants' roles. *Aphasiology, 20*(6), 483–510.

van de Sandt-Koenderman, M. (2004). High-tech AAC and aphasia; Widening horizons? *Aphasiology, 18*(3), 245–263.

Varley, R., & Whiteside, S. (2001). What is the underlying impairment in acquired apraxia of speech? *Aphasiology, 15*(1), 39–84.

Whitworth, A. B., Webster, J. M., & Howard, D. (2005). *A cognitive neuropsychological approach to assessment and intervention in aphasia: A clinician's guide.* Hove, UK: Psychology Press.

Worrall, L. (1999). *Functional communication therapy planner (FCTP).* Oxford, UK: Winslow Press.

Yoshihata, H., Watamori, T., Chujo, T., & Masuyama, K. (1998). Acquisition and generalization of mode interchange skills in people with severe aphasia. *Aphasiology, 12*, 1035–1046.

Impairment and Functional-Social Approaches for Severe Apraxia of Speech and Aphasia

Convergences and Divergences

Nina Simmons-Mackie and David Howard

The authors of the articles on impairment-oriented and social-functional treatment of severe aphasia agree on the ultimate goals of intervention. These aims of therapy are succinctly stated by Howard: "(a) the most effective communication possible, whatever the means, and (b) working with the client to maximize their ability to participate in social interactions, at any level." Dr. Howard argues that the division between "social-" and "impairment-based" approaches to aphasia therapy is not about aims, but about means or methods of achieving these aims. This statement is supported by the content of both articles.

Both authors support evidence-based practice. Howard directly calls for evidence-based methods, whereas Dr. Simmons-Mackie implies this, based on references to available research evidence to support proposed methods. Both authors agree on the need for goals to be selected based on negotiation between the therapist(s) and the client. In addition, both authors suggest similar therapy methods. Both focus on spoken expression by working on articulatory production. Howard proposes a combination of "synthetic" and "holistic" treatment of articulation; Simmons-Mackie proposes "sound production" and key word or phrase treatment. Although the terminology differs, the described methods are very similar.

Both authors propose a "total communication" approach involving training of various means of supplementing spoken communication (e.g., writing, gesture, drawing, communication booklet use, electronic devices). In addition, partner training and an aphasia group are included in recommendations for GJ by both authors.

One difference between the two articles lies in the focus of assessment. Although Simmons-Mackie mentions the need to more fully investigate motor versus linguistic deficits and the source of writing deficits, Howard details the rationale and methods of investigating underlying deficits (e.g., phonological versus motor programming basis of expressive difficulties). Although this appears to be a difference in "degree," rather than philosophy or approach, Howard's in-depth assessment is intended to lead to a more "informed" treatment of the underlying expressive impairments.

Another major difference appears to be the extent of focus on natural events and functional tasks during both assessment and treatment. Although both authors propose treatment aimed at reducing impairment and improving communication (e.g., total communication, group therapy, partner training), the social approach includes a variety of "participation"-oriented assessments and interventions that are aimed at specific aspects of GJ's life (e.g., betting on horses, visiting with family, communicating via E-mail). Also the social approach involves more functionally oriented activities such as scripts, conversation management, E-mail training, and book clubs. Methods of assessing outcomes in these areas are mentioned within the social approach, but not the impairment approach.

Although assessment of environmental barriers and supports are mentioned only in the social approach, one aspect of environmental intervention—partner training (assuming that partner skill is an aspect of the communicative environment) is recommended by both authors. The described social approach includes direct attention to GJ's psychosocial well-being and personal identity as an aspect of communication intervention. Although the description of the impairment-oriented approach includes group therapy (one means of addressing psychosocial issues), the attention to affective factors is not explicitly directed at GJ's individual needs (although there is no reason to assume such needs would be ignored in this approach).

Overall it appears that social and impairment therapy (as described by Howard and Simmons-Mackie) share common goals. Whereas some methods of assessment and intervention are shared, others differ. Impairment therapy focuses explicitly on reducing impairment and improving communication to maximize participation in social interactions. Generalization of gains to "real life," beyond those simulated in group therapy, is not addressed directly. Social-functional therapy focuses on reducing impairment and explicitly improving communication in order to maximize participation in social interactions, and focuses explicitly on engagement in life and personal affective factors to enhance carryover of gains into relevant life situations.

In cases of people with severe aphasia social- and impairment-based approaches converge. With a shared aim—the best possible communication (whatever the means)—to enable effective social participation in as many contexts as possible, the approaches differ only in their assessments and their therapy methods.

SECTION IV

10

A Case of Nonfluent Aphasia and Agrammatism

Cynthia K. Thompson and Linda Worrall

Case Description

This section addresses treatment for a gentleman with nonfluent aphasia, from two perspectives: impairment-based and client-centered, presented in Chapters 11 and 12, respectively. TC is a 62-year-old, monolingual, left-handed, English-speaking gentleman, who is 3 years postonset of aphasia, resulting from stroke. He is well educated, with bachelor's degrees in political science and biology, a master's degree in history, and a doctorate in law. Prior to his stroke he was a professor of law at a major university law school.

TC is married with two grown children and three grandchildren. His wife works full time outside the home. His son and family reside in another state, and his daughter and family live nearby. TC enjoys spending time with family and friends; he has always been an avid reader (primarily periodicals and nonfiction accounts of the civil war and other historical events). He is presently able to read John Grisham and other novels slowly (4–5 pages a day), but has difficulty reading the newspaper. He enjoys opera, the theater, and is a big fan of foreign films, although he cannot read subtitles.

Medical History

TC suffered a left-hemisphere, thromboembolic stroke in the distribution of the middle cerebral artery, which resulted in Broca's aphasia and a right upper extremity hemiparesis. Neuroimaging, using MRI, at 3 years poststroke showed a lesion involving the anterior perisylvian region, including Broca's area. He has a history of heart disease, but no prior neurological disease, psychiatric disorders, alcoholism, or developmental speech, language, or learning problems. TC passed a pure-tone screening at 500, 1000, 2000, and 4000 Hz at 30 dB binaurally. With glasses, TC's vision is 20/20. He is ambulatory.

Language Test Data

TC's performance on published tests for aphasia is listed in Table 10-1. These include the Western Aphasia Battery (WAB,; Kertesz 2006), the Boston Naming Test (Kaplan et al., 2001), the Psycholinguistic Assessment of Language Performance in Aphasia (PALPA; Kay, Lesser, & Coltheart, 1992), and the Pyramids and Palm Trees test (Howard & Patterson, 1992).

Communication Goals

The communication goals of TC include the following:

1. To participate in conversations with family and friends. TC complains that the topics are always driven by others, that he is a responder, rather than an initiator.
2. To take adult education classes in topics such as the History of Islam. TC has previously tried such courses, but he has difficulty comprehending lectures; he cannot ask questions; and he cannot take notes.
3. To expand his reading to periodicals and nonfiction books. TC complains that he cannot read newspaper headlines.
4. To read subtitles of foreign films and opera.

Table 10–1. Aphasia Test Scores

Test	Score	Test	Score
WESTERN APHASIA BATTERY			
Aphasia Quotient	78.6	**RAVEN'S COLORED MATRICES**	86%
Information Content	8/10	**BOSTON NAMING TEST**	43/60
Fluency		**PYRAMIDS AND PALM TREES TEST**	
Comprehension	4/10	Picture Association	98
Yes/No Questions	57/60	Matching	
Auditory Word Recognition	86/100	Word Association Matching	98
Sequential Commands	49/60		
Repetition	80/100	**PALPA SUBTESTS**	
Naming		***Picture and Word Semantics***	
Object Naming	53/100		
Word Fluency	14/20	Spoken Word-Picture Matching	100
Sentence Completion	10/10		
Responsive Speech	10/10	Written Word-Picture Matching	100
		Auditory Synonym	
Reading	38/40	High Imageability	100
Reading Comprehension of Sentences	20/20	Low Imageability	100
		Written Synonym	
Reading Commands	6/6	High Imageability	97
Written Word-Object Matching	6/6	Low imageability	97
		Word Semantic Association	
Written Word-Picture Matching	4/6	High Imageability	100
Spoken Word-Written Word Matching	6/6	Low Imageability	87

(continues)

Table 10–1. *(continued)*

Test	Score	Test	Score
Letter Discrimination	6/6	*Reading*	
Spelled Word Recognition	6/6	Visual Lexical Decision	100
Spelling	6/6	Oral Reading Regular and Irregular	100
Writing	20/34	Oral Reading Syllable Length	96
Writing on Request	6/10	Oral Reading Real Words	98
Written Output	10/10		
Writing to Dictation	22/22		
Writing of Dictated Words	7/7		
Alphabet and Numbers	10/10		

References

Howard, D., & Patterson, K. (1992). *Pyramids and Palm Trees*. Bury St. Edmonds, UK: Thames Valley Publishing.

Kaplan, E., Goodglass, H., & Weintraub, S. (2001). *The Boston Naming Test*. (2nd ed.). Baltimore: Lippincott, Williams and Wilkins

Kay, J., Lesser, R., & Coltheart M. (1992). *Psycholinguistic Assessment of Language Performance in Aphasia* (PALPA). East Sussex, England: Lawrence Erlbaum.

Kertesz, A. (2006). *The Western Aphasia Battery-Revised*. San Antonio, TX: Harcourt Assessment, Inc.

11

Impairment-Based Treatment for Agrammatism from a Neurolinguistic Perspective

Cynthia K. Thompson

Improving language is the primary goal of impairment-based treatment for aphasia. Although the approach does not preclude consideration of functional goals, the focus is on directly treating the deficits presented by the client. Results of testing allow the clinician to pinpoint aspects of language that are impaired and, importantly, to determine the source of the deficit to the extent possible. For example, impaired sentence production is common in nonfluent aphasia with agrammatism. However, deficit patterns vary. Some clients have syntactic deficits, others have difficulty with grammatical morphology, and many have both. Thus, tests for syntax and morphology must be included as part of the assessment battery. The data gathered then are analyzed within both psycholinguistic and cognitive neuropsychological frameworks and treatment targets are developed.

Once the impairments and their source are determined, treatment is designed. Although there are a number of approaches to impairment-based treatments, the approach recommended here is grounded by mutually supportive normal representation (formal linguistics) and language processing/production accounts. Our treatment data and that of others show that recovery of sentence production (and comprehension) "follows a path of linguistic knowledge" (Goodglass 1971; Thompson, in press). Thus, selecting treatment targets that exploit this path and result in maximal learning and generalization to untrained structures is recommended. In addition, this approach has been shown to impact functional language use (Ballard & Thompson, 1999; Jacobs 2001).

Premises Versus Promises

One of the primary premises of impairment-based treatment for agrammatism is that the aphasia represents a fractionated "normal" language system. This notion is based on the fact that agrammatism affects some, but not all, domains of language and that, within domains, all components are not equally impaired. For example, agrammatism affects primarily morphosyntactic aspects of language, and some morphosyntactic structures are often more impaired than others. However, impairment-based approaches hold that language is not lost. Rather the problem lies in *access* to language; that is, in the ability to engage the required processing routines to compute language.

Consistent with this view of aphasia, impairment-based treatment embraces the notion that treatment improves access to language. This is supported in part by observations that language recovery is systematic, rather than general, at least in chronic agrammatism. That is, when treatment is provided for certain language structures, linguistically related structures also improve with no treatment required. These observations are not surprising given recent advances in neuroscience. For example, data show that the brain is influenced by experience. It is now well established in the animal literature that motor learning, tactile and auditory stimulation affect organization of the primary motor, somatosensory, and auditory cortices, respectively (Greenough, Larson, & Withers, 1985; Recanzone, Schreiner, & Merzenich, 1993; Van Praag, Kempermann, & Gage, 1999). Studies also have shown that rehabilitative training after injury results in enhancement of representational plasticity (Nudo, Milliken, Jenkins, & Merzenich, 1996; Xerri, Merzenich, Peterson, & Jenkins, 1998), indicating that experience directly shapes physiological reorganization following brain damage. Several studies examining training-induced recovery from aphasia also indicate that treatment affects the neural networks engaged to support language (see Thompson, 2005, for review). Thus, impairment-based treatment likely improves both trained as well as untrained (linguistically related) structures because both require similar processing routines and engage similar neural mechanisms. In addition, it is noteworthy that language improvement and concomitant changes in brain mechanisms occur even in patients who are several years poststroke, indicating the malleabilitiy of the brain and language throughout the life span.

Another premise of impairment-based approaches to aphasia treatment is that functional language use will emerge as a by-product of successful treatment. Thus, the ability to participate in communication activities will result from treatment. Indeed, this is intuitive: if the impairment that precludes functional language use is ameliorated, then functional language use should improve. That is, treatment that successfully improves language ability will also positively impact functional language.

Importantly, however, these are premises, not promises, of impairment-based treatment. Intervention for agrammatism, like that for any aphasia, requires ongoing assessment of the effects of treatment, not only on trained structures, but also on untrained structures. In addition, the impact of treatment on functional language is measured. Thus, although predictions can be made about learning and generalization, nothing is assumed. If generalization does not result, the focus of the treatment is altered; it is either shifted to different structures/impairments and/or focused directly on language use in daily activities. Indeed, generalization to untrained language and to functional communication contexts is the gold standard of aphasia treatment; without it treatment may be deemed ineffective. Considering TC's language deficit profile and functional goals, Figure 11-1 demonstrates the desired flow from impairment to participation in communication activities. Clearly, neurolinguistic or other impairment-based treatments may not completely improve all levels. The figure simply shows how functional and participation goals might be impacted by improving corresponding language abilities.

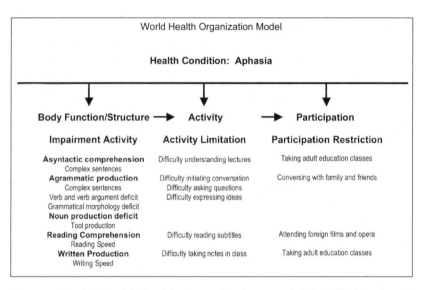

Figure 11–1. World Health Organization model detailed for treatment of TC's aphasia.

Case Interpretation

TC is a well-educated gentleman who presents with agrammatic aphasia of moderate severity, resulting from a 3-year-old stroke. He is extremely motivated to improve his language skills and has identified a number of functional goals, including the ability to be a more active participant in conversations, to be able to take adult education classes, to read periodicals and nonfiction books, and to read the subtitles of foreign films and operas. Review of language test results identifies a number of deficits that influence these communication abilities. First, his WAB profile is consistent with a diagnosis of nonfluent (Broca's) aphasia. Comprehension is superior to production, although both single word and sentence comprehension problems are evident; for example, Auditory Word Recognition and Sequential Command subtest scores are depressed. Reading comprehension, however, appears to be only mildly impaired (i.e., he scored 100% correct on all reading subtests except Reading Comprehension of Sentences [38/40] and Spoken Word-Written Word Matching [4/6]).

Production impairments are revealed by TC's WAB fluency score of 4, which is indicative of nonfluent output. Naming difficulty also is evident on the BNT (score 43/60); however, the source of the naming impairment does not appear to be related to a semantic deficit, as he performed well on both the picture and word versions of the Pyramids and Palm Trees test (Howard, & Patterson, 1992). WAB scores also show impaired Written Output and Writing to Dictation.

Additional Assessment

Initial testing reveals ample data to generate a diagnosis of nonfluent aphasia; however, it does not provide essential information required to provide optimal treatment. The WAB does not test important aspects of word and sentence production or comprehension in either spoken or written domains. Thus, additional testing in these areas is needed. For TC these include those developed in my research laboratory (the Aphasia and Neurolinguistics Research Laboratory at Northwestern University), specifically designed for examining nonfluent, agrammatic aphasia: (a) the Northwestern Assessment of Verbs and Sentences (NAVS, Thompson, in preparation), which examines verb comprehension and production, argument structure production, and comprehension and production of simple and complex sentences; (b) the Northwestern Naming Battery (NNB; Thompson & Weintraub, in preparation), which tests noun naming by semantic category and verb naming by argument structure type; (c) the Verb Inflection Test (VIT; Thompson and Bastiaanse, in preparation), which tests production of both finite and nonfinite verb forms; and (d) narrative language analysis, to evaluate TC's lexical and morphosyntactic abilities in spontaneous speech (Thompson, Shapiro, Tait, Jacobs, Schneider, & Ballard, 1995).

Data derived from administration of these measures are shown in Table 11-1. The NAVS results indicate that comprehension of syntactically complex sentences, for example, passives such as *"The man is kissed by the woman,"* and object relatives such as *"They saw the man who the woman is kissing,"* is difficult. However, simpler sentences, including actives and subject relatives are easier for TC to understand. This is a common comprehension pattern

Table 11–1. Performance on Tests of Morphosyntax and Naming, and Results of Narrative Language Analysis

Northwestern Assessment of Verbs and Sentences (NAVS)

Verb Comprehension Test	%	*Sentence Comprehension Test*	%
One-argument	100	Active	100
Two-argument	100	Passive	60
Three-argument	100	Subject Relative	100
Verb Naming Test		Object Relative	60
One-argument	7/8	Subject Wh-Questions	80
Two-argument	10/16	Object Wh-Questions	70
Three-argument	7/16	Yes/No Questions	100
Verb Argument Structure Production Test		*Sentence Production Priming Test*	
One-argument	100	Active	80
Two-argument	60	Passive	0
Three-argument	40	Subject Relative	20
		Object Relative	0
		Subject Wh-Questions	60
		Object Wh-Questions	20
		Yes/No Questions	60

Verb Inflection Test (VIT)	%	**Northwestern Naming**	
Present singular [follow_s_]	15	**Battery (NNB)**	
Present plural [follow]	25	Animals	85
Regular past [follow_ed_]	10	Fruits/Vegetables	84
Present progressive [follow_ing_]	80	Tools	40
		Clothing	65
Infinitive [to follow]	85	Low Frequency	60
Narrative Analysis			
Mean Length of Utterance	4.0		
Proportion of Grammatical Sentences	45		
Open Class/Closed Class Ratio	2.9		
Noun/Verb Ratio	3.2		
Verbs with Correct Argument Structure	44		

in agrammatism;[1] that is, canonical forms (Subject-Verb-Object, in English) are easier than noncanonical ones, likely because the latter are syntactically more complex. Given these data, it is not surprising that TC has difficulty understanding lecture material in adult-education classes as well as conversation. It also is likely that TC's comprehension deficits influence other activities that he has not specifically identified. On the NAVS Sentence Production Priming Test, production of all sentence types is compromised, with noncanonical sentences more impaired than canonical ones, suggesting a syntactic deficit in production as well.

Testing of TC's naming or word retrieval ability using the NAVS and NNB shows that, in addition to noun naming, verb naming also is impaired, and verbs are more difficult to name than nouns. Furthermore, the NAVS results show that naming verbs with a greater number of arguments are more difficult than naming those with fewer, although verb comprehension is unimpaired (NAVS verb comprehension scores show 100% correct performance across verb types). Administration of the NNB also reveals that TC's naming is better for living than nonliving things, and that tool naming is particularly difficult. Notably, problems with tool naming often coincide with verb naming deficits in aphasia (Rogalski et al., 2006). In addition, TC has the greatest difficulty naming low-frequency nouns.

Administration of the VIT, which uses action pictures and a sentence completion task to test verb inflection, shows that production of infinitive (*The dog wants to follow the cat*) and present progressive forms (*The dog is following the cat*) are unimpaired, but finite verb production is difficult for TC. Production of both present singular and plural forms, as well as past tense forms, are impaired with performance at 15%, 25%, and 10% correct, respectively (e.g., *The dog follows the cat*, *The dogs follow the cat*, *The dog followed the cat*, respectively).

Production deficits also show up in TC's spontaneous speech. Utterances are short; only 45% are grammatical sentences; he produces more open class than closed class words; and within the open class, he produces more nouns than verbs. When verbs are produced, verb arguments are missing from the discourse. These findings show

---

[1]Some agrammatic speakers do not show this pattern (see Berndt et al., 1996).

production deficits that, not surprisingly, impair TC's ability to initiate conversational topics, ask questions in classroom situations, and to express his thoughts and ideas in other situations as well.

Finally, the *Gates-MacGinitie Reading Tests* (Gates & MacGinitie, 1965), administered to examine reading comprehension, speed, and accuracy, show comprehension of words and paragraphs near ceiling. However, TC's reading speed is slow.

Treatment Goals

The overall goal of treatment is to improve access to language by focusing on impairments revealed by the language evaluation. Generalization from trained to untrained structures and to functional language serve as the primary outcome measures. Based on TC's data, treatment goals will be to improve spoken and written sentence comprehension and production. Additional goals concerned with processing speed in listening and reading also are prescribed. Specific goals are to (a) improve spoken and written comprehension and production of complex syntactic forms, (b) improve spoken and written production of verbs with complex argument structure entries, (c) improve spoken and written production of finite verb forms, and (d) increase both oral reading and reading comprehension speed.

Functional goals for TC will be to improve (a) comprehension of real-time speech while listening in conversation, lectures, and other venues; (b) comprehension of written text in books, periodicals, and other material, (c) ability to express ideas and ask questions in group conversations, classrooms, and other settings, and (d) expression of ideas in writing.

Treatment

A neurolinguistic treatment approach is recommended (Goodglass 1971; Jakobson 1964; Lesser 1978; Murray, Timberlake, & Eberle, 2007; Thompson, Shapiro, Ballard, Jacobs, Schneider, & Tait, 1997, Thompson, Shapiro, Kiran, & Sobecks, 2003). This approach exploits what is known about normal language representation and processing and controls relevant linguistic variables in selection of structures entered into treatment and for development of the treatment itself. For example, sentences trained are controlled for both lexical and syntactic variables and treatment emphasizes sentence formation. The verbs used in treatment are selected based on their argument structure and the thematic roles that they assign. For example, some verbs such as *sleep* assign only one argument, an Agent, whereas others assign two or three, for example, *follow* and *send*, respectively. Syntactic structures are selected based on their linguistic properties, and grammatical morphemes are selected based on their morphosyntactic features.

Language structures trained are chosen to maximize generalization to untrained structures. Research has indicated two important variables related to generalization: (a) generalization occurs to linguistically related, but not unrelated, structures, and (b) generalization is enhanced when the direction of treatment is from *more* to *less* complex structures. Crucially, the latter occurs only when complex and simple structures are linguistically related to one another (Thompson, 2007). The *Complexity Account of Treatment Efficacy* (CATE) states that: "training complex structures results in generalization to less complex structures when untreated structures encompass processes relevant to . . . treated ones" (Thompson et al., 2003, p. 602). This effect has been shown in treating both sentence production/comprehension and naming in aphasia (Kiran 2007; Thompson & Shapiro 2007) as well as in treating language and phonological disorders in children (see Gierut, 2007). Linguistically related structures are selected for training and a complexity hierarchy is established for them based on their linguistic properties. If property Y is encompassed within property X, then training X should result in generalization to Y. But, because this is a unidirectional relationship, training Y should have no effect on X.

Complexity hierarchies differ depending on the language domain treated. Complexity in the syntactic domain considers the syntactic properties of sentences, including the order in which elements appear in sentences (i.e., canonical vs. noncanonical word order), the types of phrasal movement involved in generating the sentence form, and the number of propositions and embedded clauses. In the area of word comprehension or production, the linguistic relation among words is considered, including grammatical class. For example, verbs and nouns belong to different grammatical classes so generalization from one to the other would not be expected.

Lexical variables within each class also are considered. For verbs, both the number and type of arguments selected by the verb and semantic variables (such as motion or change of state) enter into the equation; and for nouns semantic categories as well as the relation among elements within the category are considered. For example, Kiran and Thompson (2003) developed complexity hierarchies based on prototypicality (i.e., extent to which the semantic features of items within a category are similar to or different from the category prototype).

The neurolinguistic approach uses metalinguistic strategies to train selected language structures. That is, processes assumed to underlie sentence and word production and comprehension are emulated. In sentence training, phrase structure building operations are practiced, for example, verb and verb argument selection, placement of sentence constituents in word strings to form simple sentence frames, and movement of constituents to form complex, noncanonical forms.

Importantly, even though the neurolinguistic approach aims to improve morphosyntactic aspects of language, care is taken when selecting the vocabulary included in target structures. For TC low-frequency nouns and tool names are particularly difficult; thus, including these in target sentences, where appropriate, is recommend. In addition, functionally relevant vocabulary is selected. For TC, vocabulary relevant to history, politics, movies, theatre, opera, and his family would be used, including both common and proper nouns (e.g., names of family members, friends, political figures, films). Furthermore, both individual and group treatment sessions are part of this approach. In individual sessions explicit rule-based treatment is provided and in group sessions functional goals are addressed by emphasizing the use of trained language in group settings and in simulated environments in the clinic. In addition, conversational partners are provided with information about aphasia in general and how best to communicate with aphasic people. Treatment targets also are shared with family members so that the latter can be practiced at home.

Sentence Comprehension and Production Treatment

Treatment focused on noncanonical sentences with syntactic movement, both Wh-movement and NP-movement, is recommended for

TC. (Wh- and NP-movement are linguistic constructs that address the derivation of complex sentences; see Thompson, in press, for review.). In keeping with CATE, this involves direct training of the most complex sentences and testing generalization to structures of lesser complexity. Consider the following sentences, which involve Wh-movement, listed from more to less complex:

1. The judge watched the defendant who the witness framed. (object relative)
2. It was the pianist who the conductor called. (object cleft)
3. What country did the U.S. military invade? (object wh-question)

When training Wh-movement, object relative structures (1 above) would be trained first with generalization tested to object cleft structures and wh-questions, (2 and 3 above, respectively), as well as simple active forms (*The professor watched the debate team*). NP-movement training would target subject-raising structures, such as in (4), as generalization is tested to passives sentences as in (5):

4. The governor seems to have canceled the meeting.
5. The president was guarded by the secret service.

Importantly, all sentences are constructed with multisyllabic, low-frequency nouns and two-argument verbs, which are intermixed across sentence types. Treatment of Underlying Forms (TUF) is recommended for training both auditory and reading comprehension as well as spoken sentence production (see Thompson, in press; Thompson & Shapiro, 2005, for details).

Treatment of Auditory and Reading Comprehension Speed

TC's case history and test data indicate that auditory and reading comprehension speed are slow. Therefore, treatment targeting processing speed using the same structures discussed above is suggested. For auditory comprehension, simple scenarios and yes/no probe questions would be developed. The speed of presentation of the scenarios would be systematically increased, for example, from 60 to 140 words per minute. For example, TC will listen to a scenario such as:

> This is the story of a modern opera. The main characters are a dictator, the dictator's brother, Richard, and an assassin. The dictator paid the assassin to murder Richard. But, the assassin murdered the dictator instead. Richard was relieved.
>
> *Probe:* "It was the dictator who(m) the assassin murdered". (yes/no)

Treatment aimed to improve reading comprehension, as is required for reading opera and foreign film subtitles, would proceed in a similar manner. However, scenarios would be broken down into lines of text, consisting of two sentences each. Text lines would then be presented on a computer screen with presentation duration decreased systematically (e.g., from 60 to 15 seconds) across trials. Probe questions (i.e., yes/no) would be interjected between text lines, with the number of lines presented between probes increasing (from two to five) across trials. A sample scenario, with probes presented following every two text lines, follows:

> The dictator expects a revolution. He talks to his brother, Richard. The dictator suspects that Richard is plotting the revolution. He accuses Richard.
>
> *Probe:* Did the dictator expect a revolution?
>
> The dictator makes a plan. He finds an assassin to murder his brother. The dictator trusts that the assassin will do the job. He pays the assassin.
>
> *Probe:* Did the dictator find an assassin?
>
> The assassin suspects a problem. The assassin investigates the situation. The assassin learns that Richard is innocent. The assassin is clever.
>
> *Probe:* Did the assassin think that Richard is guilty?
>
> The assassin finds Richard. The assassin and Richard talk through the night.
> The assassin makes a plan. The assassin will murder the dictator.

Probe: Did the assassin talk to Richard?

The assassin meets the dictator. He gives the dictator a poison drink. The dictator is dizzy; he stumbles and falls. The assassin walks away.

Probe: Did the assassin push the dictator?

Treatment of Verbs Controlled for Argument Structure Complexity

For verb treatment, complexity hierarchies based on verb argument structure would be developed. Verb arguments are the participant roles that are entailed by the verb, for example, the person performing an action (i.e., the Agent) and the person or things that are acted upon (i.e., the Theme). Research has shown that verbs with two and three arguments are more difficult to produce than one-argument verbs (Jonkers & Bastiaanse, 1998; Kim & Thompson, 2000, 2004; Luzzatti et al., 2002, and others). For example, verbs like *send* or *donate* have three arguments (see [1] below); verbs like *kiss* or *follow* have two arguments (see [2] below) and verbs like *smile* or *whisper* have only one argument (see [3] below).

1. The scholar *donated* the collection to the library.
   The professor *sent* the manuscript to the publisher.
2. The composer *kissed* the producer.
   The photographer *followed* the celebrities.
3. The president elect *smiled*.
   The attorney general *whispered*.

In addition, verbs with arguments that do not directly map onto sentence positions are difficult for persons with agrammatic aphasia. One-argument verbs like *fall* and *melt*, called unaccusatives, have a Theme argument in the subject position, rather than an Agent as in *smile* and *whisper*. This situation results from movement of the Theme (which usually is in the object position in sentences) to the subject position (cf. *The empire fell; The glacier melted.* versus *The president smiled; The general whispered*). Similarly, some psychological (psych) verbs, defined as verbs that require an Experiencer argument, have a simple mapping of the Experiencer argument onto the subject position, as in the verbs *admire* and *fear* (e.g., <u>*The soldiers*</u> *admired the captain*; <u>*The explorers*</u> *feared the lightning*). However, other psych verbs involve special syntactic operations and/or semantic features that place the Experiencer in the object position, such as *amuse* and *frighten* (e.g., *The captain amused* <u>*the soldiers*</u>; *The lightning frightened* <u>*the explorers*</u>). These operations/features render the latter more complex than the former, and therefore they are more difficult to produce (see Lee & Thompson, 2003). Treatment targeting more complex verbs such as three-argument verbs, unaccusative and Experiencer-type psych verbs is recommended, with generalization tested to less complex verbs. Importantly, verbs should be trained in sentence contexts and a modified TUF approach can be used, focused on both comprehension and production of verbs and verb arguments, as well as any movement required to generate surface sentence forms. Both written and spoken production would be trained.

In addition, in the written modality, treatment would focus on strategies for note taking, teaching TC to extract the verb and certain arguments from auditory sentences. For example, a target sentence using the two-argument verb "defeat" might be: "Western nations defeated the Ottoman Empire." In the first phase of treatment TC would hear such sentences and be required to identify and write (a) the action word, *defeat*, (b) what was defeated, and (c) who did the defeating, and to generate complete sentences. Next, he would practice identifying constituents required to write when taking notes. Practice using a digital tape recorder and computer also would be provided. The clinician would read sentences and short paragraphs for TC to record, enter into the computer, and edit by extracting relevant verbs and other key material.

Treating Grammatical Morphology

Another problem for TC is producing grammatical morphemes, particularly tense and agreement markers. Thus, treatment needs to address this. Specifically, treatment on regular past tense, third person singular, and third person plural (see sentences below) is recommended.

The journalist fil*ed* the evidence. (regular past)
The journalist file*s* the evidence. (third person singular)
The journalist*s* fil*e* the evidence. (third person plural)

Predicting patterns of generalization from tense to agreement or from agreement to tense is difficult because there is debate in the linguistic literature with regard to how these elements are related to one another. On some linguistic accounts (see Pollock, 1989), tense is considered to be more difficult than agreement because tense is projected from a higher node than agreement in the syntactic tree (i.e., the Tree Pruning Hypothesis suggests this; Friedmann & Grodzinsky, 1998). However, other accounts propose that they are projected from the same node (Bobaljik & Thrainsson, 1998). Still others, which consider the featural detail of tense and agreement, suggest that agreement is more complex than tense. In fact, in a recent study, we found that training agreement improved tense for many participants, but the opposite pattern was seen in only a few (Thompson, Milman, Dickey, O'Connor, Arcuri, & Choy, 2006). Given these differing accounts, CATE makes no specific prediction regarding the direction of generalization between tense and agreement markers, even though the two are linguistically related. Simultaneous targeting of all structures is, therefore, recommended. This would involve training grammatical encoding, using temporal adverbs (e.g., *yesterday, everyday*), and grammatical morpheme selection. This would be followed by practice with insertion of sentential elements into sentence frames and thematic role training.

Outcome Measures

To evaluate treatment efficacy, I recommend developing probe measures established to test both trained and untrained structures periodically throughout and at the end of treatment. In addition, both narrative and conversational discourse samples are important to collect and analyze for (a) morphosyntactic and lexical variables, and (b) content and efficiency of communication (after Thompson et al., 1995 and Nicholas & Brookshire, 1993, respectively). Narrative samples are collected by asking TC to describe familiar movies, operas, and events; conversational discourse is sampled with both familiar and unfamiliar conversational partners discussing various topics (see Thompson et al., 1995, for data collection details and results of linguistic coding of narrative and conversational dyads). The Gates-MacGinitie Reading Test also could be administered to evaluate changes in reading speed. This test includes alternative forms, which makes it useful for evaluation of reading ability over time.

Monitoring language periodically during group treatment and in functional settings also is recommended. This includes evaluation of both linguistic and communicative variables.

Summary

This chapter describes an impairment-based approach for treatment of TC's agrammatic aphasia, emphasizing access to grammatical forms that are difficult for him. Treatment methods capitalize on what is known about normal language representation and processing as well as research that has charted morphosyntactic recovery patterns in agrammatism. The approach controls the structural complexity of both lexical and morphosyntactic variables in selection of treatment targets, and treatment stresses sentence structure building operations, from lexical selection to placement of constituents in sentence frames.

Promoting maximal generalization to untrained language structures is at the heart of neurolinguistic treatment. Although generalized use of language in functional situations is the ultimate goal of treatment, rather than directly treating functional skills, neurolinguistic treatment aims to improve language itself. Throughout treatment the impact of improved language on daily communication activities is evaluated and strategies for using language in these contexts are provided. If or when generalization to functional contexts is not accomplished or is incomplete, treatment is extended to group or other functional situations.

References

Ballard, K. J., & Thompson, C. K. (1999). Treatment and generalization of complex sentence structures in agrammatism. *Journal of Speech, Language, and Hearing Research, 42,* 690–707.

Bobaljik, J., & Thrainsson, H. (1988). Two heads aren't always better than one. Syntax, 1(1), 37–71.

Friedmann, N.,, & Grodzinsky, Y. (1997). Tense and agreement in agrammatic production: Pruning the syntactic tree. *Brain and Language, 56*(3), 397–425.

Gates, A. I., & MacGinitie, W. H. (1965). *Gates-MacGinitie Reading Tests.* New York: Teachers College Press.

Gierut, J. (2007). Phonological complexity and language learnability. *American Journal of Speech and Language Pathology, 6,* 6-17.

Goodglass, H. (1971). Agrammatism. In H. Whitaker, & H. Whitaker (Eds.), *Perspectives in neurolinguistics and psycholinguistics* (pp. 237-259). New York: Academic Press.

Greenough, W., Larson, J., & Withers, G. (1985). Effects of unilateral and bilateral training in a reaching task on dendritic branching of neurons in the rat motor sensory forelimb cortex. *Behavioral Neural Biology, 44,* 301-314.

Howard, D., & Patterson, K. E. (1992). *Pyramids and Palm Trees test.* Edmunds, UK: Thames Valley Test Company.

Jacobs, B. (2001). Social validity of changes in informativeness and efficiency of aphasic discourse following linguistic specific treatment (LST). *Brain and Language, 78,* 115-127.

Jakobson, R. (1964). Toward a linguistic typology of aphasic impairments. In A. V. S. de Reuck & M. O'Connor (Eds.), *Disorders of language* (pp. 21-42). London: Churchill Livingstone.

Kaplan, E., Goodglass, H., & Weintraub, S. (2001). *Boston Naming Test* (2nd ed.). Philadelphia: Lippincott Williams & Wilkins.

Kay, J., Lesser, R., & Coltheart, M . (1992). *Psycholinguistic assessments of language processing in aphasia.* New York: Psychology Press.

Kim, M., & Thompson, C. K. (2000). Patterns of comprehension and production of nouns and verbs in agrammatism: Implications for lexical organization. *Brain and Language, 74,* 1-25.

Kim, M., & Thompson, C. K. (2004). Verb deficits in Alzheimer's disease and agrammatism: Implications for lexical organization. *Brain and Language, 88,* 1-20.

Kiran, S. (2007). Complexity in the treatment of naming deficits. *American Journal of Speech and Language Pathology, 16,* 18-29.

Kiran, S., & Thompson, C. K. (2003). Effects of exemplar typicality on naming in aphasia. *Journal of Speech, Language, and Hearing Research, 46,* 608-622.

Lee, M., & Thompson, C. K. (2003). Agrammatic aphasic production and comprehension of unaccusative verbs in sentence contexts. *Journal of Neurolinguistics, 17,* 315-330.

Lesser, R. (1978). *Linguistic investigations of aphasia.* New York: Elsevier.

Luzzatti, C., Raggi, R., Zonca, G., Pistarini, C., Contardi, A., & Pinna, G. D. (2002). Verb-noun double dissociation in aphasic lexical impairments: The role of word frequency and imageability. *Brain and Language, 81,* 432-444.

Murray, L., Timberlake, A., & Eberle, R. (2007). Treatment of underlying forms in a discourse context. *Aphasiology, 21,* 139-163.

Musso, M., Weiller, C., Kiebel, S., Muller, S., Bulau, P., & Rijntjes, M. (1999). Training-induced brain plasticity in aphasia. *Brain, 122,* 1781-1790.

Nicholas, L., & Brookshire, R. (1993). A system for quantifying the informativeness and efficiency of connected speech in adults with aphasia. *Journal of Speech and Hearing Research,* 36, 338-350.

Nudo, R., Milliken, G., Jenkins, W., & Merzenich, M. (1996). Neural substrates for the effects of rehabilitate training on motor recovery after ischemic infarct. *Science, 171,* 1791-1794.

Recanzone, G., Schreiner, C., & Merzenich, M. (1993). Plasticity in the frequency representation of the primary auditory cortex following discrimination training in adult owl monkeys. *Journal of Neuroscience, 13,* 87-103.

Rogalski, E., Milman, L., O'Connor, J., Medina, J., Weintraub, S., & Thompson, C. K. (2006). *Category-specific and word-class naming patterns in primary progressive aphasia.* Presentation at the 5th International FTD Conference. San Francisco, CA.

Small, S., Flores, D., & Noll, D. (1998). Different neural circuits subserve reading before and after therapy for acquired dyslexia. *Brain and Language, 62,* 298-308.

Thompson, C. K. (2005). Plasticity of language networks. In M. Baudry, X. Bi, & S. S. Schrieber (Eds.), *Syntaptic plasticity: Basic mechanisms to clinical applications* (pp. 343-355). New York: Marcel Dekker.

Thompson, C. K. (2007). Complexity in language learning and treatment. *American Journal of Speech and Language Pathology, 16,* 3-5.

Thompson, C. K. (in press). Treatment of syntactic and morphological deficits in aphasia: Treatment of underlying forms. In: R. Chapey (Ed.), *Language intervention strategies in adult aphasia* (5th ed.). Baltimore: Williams & Wilkins.

Thompson, C. K. (in preparation). *Northwestern Assessment of Verbs and Sentences.*

Thompson, C. K., Milman, L. H., Dickey, M. W., O'Connor, J. E., Bonakdarpour, B., Fix, S. C., Choy, J. J., & Arcuri, D. F. (2006). Functional category production in agrammatism: Treatment and generalization effects. *Brain and Language, 99,* 79-81.

Thompson, C. K., & Shapiro, L. P. (2007). Complexity in treatment of syntactic deficits. *American Journal of Speech and Language Pathology, 16,* 30-42.

Thompson, C. K., Shapiro, L., Ballard, K., Jacobs, B., Schneider, S. & Tait, M. (1997). Training and generalized production of wh- and NP-movement structures in agrammatic speakers. *Journal of Speech, Language and Hearing Research,* 40, 228-244.

Thompson, C. K., Shapiro, L., Kiran, S., & Sobecks, J. (2003). The role of syntactic complexity in treatment of sentence deficits in agrammatic aphasia: The complexity account of treatment efficacy (CATE). *Journal of Speech, Language, and Hearing Research, 42,* 690–707.

Thompson, C. K., Shapiro, L., Tait, M., Jacobs, B., Schneider, S., & Ballard, K. (1995). A system for the linguistic analysis of agrammatic language production. *Brain and Language, 51,* 124–127.

Thompson, C., & Weintraub, S. (in preparation). *The Northwestern Naming Battery.*

Van Praag, H., Kempermann, G., & Gage, F. (1999). Running increases cell proliferation and neurogenesis in the adult mouse dentate gyrus. *Nature Neuroscience, 2,* 266–270.

Xerri, C., Merzenich, M., Peterson, B., & Jenkins, W. (1998). Plasticity of primary somatosensory cortex paralleling sensorimotor skill recovery from stroke in adult monkeys. *Journal of Neurophysiology, 79,* 2119–2148.

12

Intervention for Agrammatism from a Consequences Perspective

Linda E. Worrall

The intervention approach described here is a client-driven approach, rather than a purely functional or consequences approach. A client-driven, rather than therapist-driven approach, works hard to establish the goals of the client and then a collaborative or shared decision-making process jointly determines the nature of the intervention, including how success should be measured. It does not assume that the goals of the client are impairment based (e.g., I want to talk better) or functional (e.g., I want to go back to work) as it assumes that every individual with aphasia will not only have a different impairment but also different lives that the aphasia must fit into. Some people with aphasia may wish to focus entirely on functional outcomes, others may want their language back and want to improve their language, and others, probably the majority, may want a combination of both.

The ICF conceptual framework (Figure 12–1) is useful to describe the broad range of goals that clients may articulate. The conceptual framework also helps to trigger the therapists' ideas about therapy strategies as some forms of intervention may be better suit-

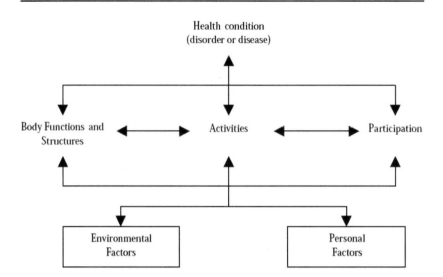

Figure 12–1. The conceptual framework of World Health Organization's International Classification of Functioning, Disability, and Health (ICF).

ed to the targets of intervention. For example, incorporating group therapy into the client's program is probably better suited to increasing social participation than individual therapy alone. The conceptual framework of the ICF also makes the relationship between components explicit. Thus, if the goal is in the Activity/Participation domain, then interventions in the surrounding Impairment and Contextual areas can have an impact on it. Interventions that directly address the Activity/Participation component are also a method of achieving the goals.

In rehabilitation for TC, interventions at all levels of the ICF are described, even though TC's goals are Activity and Participation goals. This is a departure from the traditional bottom-up rehabilitation approach, which operates on the premise that rehabilitation at the Impairment level will positively impact functional communication. The traditional rehabilitation approach also does not usually consider that increased Activity or Participation improves Impairment although there is increasing evidence to suggest that this is the case (Worrall & Yiu, 2000). Until recently, it also has not been considered that removing barriers in the environment to increase participation is within the scope of rehabilitation, yet the primary thrust of most disability legislation such as the Americans with Disability Act of 1990 has been to enhance the environment to increase participation. Professional associations such as the American Speech-Language and Hearing Association have described rehabilitation at the Environmental Factor level as a part of its Scope of Practice; therefore, speech-language pathologists are encouraged to work through all components of the ICF.

In the same way that the client does not live in a vacuum, the services that can be provided need to be contextualized as they are often constrained by finances, policies, or therapist or organizational preference. Persons with aphasia, like TC, are seen in the university clinic at The University of Queensland (UQ), Australia, which offers a 2-hour session (1 hour individual therapy, 1 hour group therapy) provided by student therapists supervised by a qualified speech pathologist (usually a staff member or a Ph.D. student) once a week for each 12-week semester. A nominal fee is paid for the block (12 weeks) of therapy (see Worrall, Davidson, Howe, & Rose, [2007] for a more detailed description of the group therapy that is provided at The University of Queensland). In addition, a therapist does not live in a vacuum. Therefore, I have purposively used personal pronouns to denote my context and individuality as a therapist. This is consistent with qualitative research paradigms that are often used in this research area.

Case Interpretation

This case of a well-educated older man with a nonfluent aphasia is typical of many referrals to the university clinic. The key features of the case description in priority order are (1) the goals of the client, (2) his personal details, and (3) the type, severity, and time post-onset of his language impairment. The important details of each of these areas follow.

1. Goals

It is noteworthy that all four goals expressed by TC are highly specific, contextualized to his life, and classified as Activity or Participation goals in the ICF. These goals serve as the starting point for treatment. This suggests that the therapist has encouraged TC to think about his communication goals and has spent time faithfully recording the specificity of the goals. That is, the therapist has not assumed that the client just wants to "talk better." It recognizes that the client has considerable insight and expertise into how aphasia has affected his life. I would further probe these goals in the first "assessment" session with the client.

2. Personal Details

TC is a highly educated man with a supportive family. There are very positive signs that he still participates in many life activities such as watching operas and foreign films, reading, and conversing with family and friends. His desire for learning has not abated with his aphasia, as he states that adult education classes on Islam are a priority for him.

3. Type, Severity, and Time Postonset of His Language Impairment

TC's WAB profile is consistent with a diagnosis of Broca's aphasia and his Aphasia Quotient (AQ) of 78.6 suggests a moderate severity. Most significantly, he is 3 years poststroke and his communication goals indicate a man who is keen to continue with his life goals. The type and severity of his language impairment are not seen as significant barriers to achieving those goals.

Additional Assessment and Treatment Goals

Assessment has many purposes including screening, diagnosis, therapy planning, and outcome measurement. The two main aims for TC's assessment are therapy planning and outcome measurement as the diagnosis of aphasia has been made and any diagnostics into specific language impairments is not necessary to achieve his goals at this stage. Indeed, most assessment results presented in the case description are not necessary for the therapy planned here. This type of assessment would only be needed if the client had specific impairment-based goals such as wanting to say little words, being able to talk in sentences, or being able to write grammatically correct sentences. A fully operational language processing system is not a prerequisite for achieving TC's goals, but a better functioning system may help.

Outcome measurement is another purpose of assessment in this case and I would seek to provide feedback that the client wishes by measuring performance on his stated goals. My preferred method is Goal Attainment Scaling (Kiresuk & Sherman, 1968; Worrall, 2000) in which progress on the client's own goals is measured. This individualized approach has many advantages, and although some clients may still wish to be assessed using standardized measures, there is a lack of appropriate measures available to examine all components of the ICF. It is more likely that TC will want to track his progress on reading the latest nonfiction book rather than the reading subtests of the PALPA or rating his enjoyment of conversation with family and friends rather than undertake the tasks of a CADL-2. He may, however, choose to be measured using standardized assessments as well as goal attainment scaling and this option would be discussed with him.

Further assessment would occur over two sessions. An entire session would be given to setting further goals and targets. The amount of time devoted to this indicates its importance within a client-driven approach.

Session 1. Initial Interview

My first and primary interest is the client's goals. The clinician needs to understand these in considerable depth and detail. It is important to determine the client's goals by asking the client about his current concerns and priorities, trying to steer away from any preconceived ideas about the type of services a speech-language pathologist may offer. Direct questions such as "What are your goals of therapy?" are too restricted to what clients think speech-language pathologist can provide. Rather, asking TC to tell the story of his stroke and aphasia and seeking to understand the context of TC's expressed communication goals are more useful. What are his current life goals and how do these communication goals help achieve them? Has he had previous therapy and how has this influenced his current goals? What did he like and dislike about his previous experiences of therapy? It also is important to seek clarification of his expressed goals and ask him to rank them in order of importance to his life.

Using the process of Goal Attainment Scaling, TC and I would talk through his goals together and work out what would be the most successful outcome for each goal and then what would be considered lesser outcomes for each goal. The prognosis for successful treatment in this case is considered excellent because TC is a highly educated man who appears to have easily defined his communication goals. An example of this goal attainment process would be:

Goal 1: To participate in group conversation with family and friends. TC complains that the topics of conversations are always driven by others; that he is a responder, rather than an initiator:

TC may suggest that the most successful outcome would be to be able to initiate conversation on at least one occasion during all group conversations with family and friends within the next 12 weeks. A lesser outcome may be that he is only able to initiate at least one topic in a group conversation with close family.

Goal 2: To take adult education classes in topics such as the History of Islam. TC has previously tried such courses, but he has difficulty comprehending lectures; he cannot ask questions; and he cannot take notes.

This goal needs to broken down and explored more fully before goal attainment takes place. Is his real goal to complete the course, or is it to independently listen to lectures, ask questions, or take notes unaided? If it is to complete and learn from the course, no matter what it takes, then it would be necessary to seek information about any disability support policies available in the adult education school on making classes accessible to all. TC may therefore be open to asking for a buddy to take notes, and asking the lecturer if the lectures could be recorded and whether he could ask the lecturer questions at the end of the lecture after the rest of the class has left. That is, before this goal can be developed into targets, additional information is needed to understand TC's motives and his attitude toward enabling support.

Goal 3: To expand his reading to periodicals and nonfiction books

Again knowing the end goal is necessary to develop a treatment plan. Is TC's goal to understand the content of the periodicals and the nonfiction books, to read for sustained periods of time, or to conquer the challenge of reading to his former ability? Some insight into what TC would consider success for this goal would depend upon probing in this area.

Goal 4: To read subtitles of foreign films and opera.

Is his final goal to enjoy opera and foreign films, to be able to get the gist of the subtitles, or effortlessly and quickly read every word in the subtitles? Each would mean that a different level of success is articulated by TC in the Goal Attainment Process.

After understanding the context of TC's goals and understanding his motives more fully, the following options would be presented. Evidence for each of the options also would be offered, so that joint decision-making is an informed process.

1. Attend weekly clinic, which has both individual therapy and a group therapy for support and practice in achieving his goals. Group therapy would only be offered if he were interested in joining a group, but the results of a randomized controlled trial (Elman, 2007; Elman & Bernstein-Ellis, 1999; Ross, Winslow, Marchant, & Brumfitt, 2006) found that group therapy was effective in improving everyday communication and conversational skills which are congruent with his goals.

2. If he also wishes to regain his former language and reading skills, attending another group that uses a cognitive neuropsychological or impairment-based approach would be suggested. At UQ, different clinics offer different treatment approaches and clients move between the clinics. From his test results, therapy may focus on sentence production skills, maybe in conjunction with some sentence comprehension work and phonological encoding treatment. Some generalization of these skills to the client-driven therapy that I provide would likely occur and the behaviors trained in the impairment-based clinic could be incorporated into his client-driven therapy. For example, if sentence comprehension was being targeted in the impairment-based therapy, then we would aim to seek to ensure that sentence comprehension checks and coaching in natural conversations occurred. For example, if I were assisting TC with his lectures about Islam then I would ask TC some comprehension questions at the end of the lecture (e.g., How did Islam spread to other parts of the world from its origins in Arabia?). TC would be informed that there is a high level of

evidence for the impairment-based approach, particularly if there is intensive practice (Basso, 2005). TC therefore would have the option of pursuing both an impairment and functional approach in The UQ clinics.

3. TC would be informed about the Australian Aphasia Association and its activities and provided with written information about the association. There is no evidence for the benefits of joining a consumer support group for people with aphasia; however, there is some evidence that attending a residential seminar with other people with aphasia is beneficial to well-being (Hinckley & Packard, 2001). It would be suggested that TC could attend or even present at the Aphasia Association's annual conference.

4. Contacting a member of the Association who is also a Professor and has offered to be a contact or buddy for any new members of the Association also would be suggested.

5. Influencing awareness of aphasia in his immediate community would be emphasized and enabling his conversational partners to be more accommodating to his communicative behavior would be highlighted. For example, his family and friends could allow TC more time to initiate topics in a group conversation. He may choose to be his own advocate, invite family and friends along to a group session at the university clinic, or recruit members of the Australian Aphasia Association to help him influence others. These are options that I would discuss with him.

Session 2. Individual Session—Measuring Baselines

A baseline for each goal then would be measured. These measures would have been discussed with TC as part of our first session on goal and target setting.

Goal 1

For his first goal, TC would be asked to keep a structured diary of his group conversations (participants, topics, duration, and the number of times he was able to initiate a conversation) during the following week. The self-report of number of times he initiated conversation per minutes of conversation would be the key baseline measure; however, it might be expected that the number and type of conversational partners and duration of conversations may increase as well. He may also be asked about the possibility of obtaining a baseline video recording of a typical group conversation from his everyday life. He then could record the number of times he initiated conversation per minutes of conversation and identify what factors might be making it more difficult for him to initiate topics. The clinician would view segments of the videotape with TC and a family member to see if they could identify what was happening. This may prompt them to suggest possible solutions.

Goal 2

After the first session, I would have spoken with the adult education lecturer who had a previous student with a learning disability who struggled with comprehending lectures, asking questions, and taking notes. He was also aware of the educational institution's disability policy. He offered TC his own lecture notes and was open to TC recording his lectures. He also suggested that TC remain after the lecture so that they could talk about the lecture and TC could ask his questions. The agreed plan was that TC was to receive the lecturer's notes the week before and read them through in preparation for the lecture, and then remain behind to discuss the lecture. If TC still struggled with the content of the lecture, then he could try video-recording the lecture with a small camcorder. It was also suggested that TC attempt to use his topic initiation skills in discussion with fellow students. The baseline would be TC's comprehension of the first lecture. Ideally, the clinician would go along to the same lecture and check TC's comprehension by asking him to demonstrate his understanding of several key points of the lecture after the class. Twenty questions about key points in the lecture would be ideal. TC and the clinician would then meet with the lecturer to discuss the accessibility plan.

Goal 3

For the third goal of being able to comprehend periodicals and nonfiction books, the baseline would be a set of comprehension questions from one of his current books or periodicals. Twenty comprehension questions would be chosen.

Goal 4

The final baseline would test his comprehension of subtitles from a rented foreign film or opera of his choice. Again, 20 comprehension questions would be chosen.

Group Session—Choice of Topics for Groups or Group Project

Groups at UQ usually consist of four to six people with aphasia who have similar goals. Like the individual sessions above, the first group session is also a goal-setting discussion. Examples of some of the goals for groups include understanding more about aphasia and stroke and educating people about aphasia. TC may find that other people in the group have attended adult education classes or also have similar difficulties and have some suggestions to offer. TC may also find people with similar interests in the group. Baseline measures for the group may involve testing their current knowledge about stroke and aphasia by a questionnaire such as that used by the National Aphasia Association (http://www.aphasia.org) or by simply asking each person to say or write down what they know about aphasia or stroke and count the number of key information units. Measures of self-efficacy (Lorig, Stewart, Ritter, Gonzalez, Laurent, & Lynch, 1996) may also be relevant here as may measures of topic initiation such as the Conversational Analysis Profile for People with Aphasia (CAPPA) (Whitworth, Perkins, & Lesser, 1997).

Treatment(s) and Outcome Measures

The manner in which TC's stated goals were refined in the first individual session and how Goal Attainment Scaling is used to drive baseline assessment were discussed above. Group therapy goal setting and assessment also are included as part of the service provision. The next section assumes that the mutually agreed goals and proposed strategies are "owned" by both TC and I and that they are subject to change. The third session of contact is now described and then a general outline of group therapy and future therapy is proposed.

Session 3. Individual Therapy

Goal 1: Initiating Conversation

Scripts for initiating conversations would be rehearsed. Other conversational partners would also be encouraged to leave TC with enough time and opportunity to initiate conversations (Hopper, Holland, & Rewega, 2002). Maintenance of turn-taking would also be addressed. Strategies are introduced in the individual session and rehearsed and coached in the group sessions. It is anticipated that some conversational partner training (Kagan, Black, Duchan, Simmons-Mackie, & Square, 2001) may have also occurred as part of the group therapy.

Goal 2: Adult Education Classes

Any problems that have arisen since commencing the adult education classes would be brainstormed with the aim of helping TC to identify and resolve some of the difficulties he is having. As a Professor of Law, TC would be well aware of the acts that legislate against disability discrimination. TC may not think of aphasia as a disability; therefore, some discussion with him about theories or models of disability may be useful.

Goal 3: Reading Periodicals and Nonfiction

If TC attends the other clinic in which the reading impairment is the focus of attention, then some work in this area may be undertaken here; but it appears from the case description that fatigue and working memory may also be factors. People with aphasia often complain that once they have understood a paragraph, they have forgotten the previous paragraph. Some clients find that reading with a ruler or using a moving frame for each line helps eliminate the distraction of the rest of the paragraph. Reading aloud may also help or highlighting keywords with a highlighter pen (particularly in periodicals) is a frequently used tool to aid comprehension. The concept of gradually increasing the amount read each day is also helpful. The concept of creating an aphasia-friendly reading environment is also important. TC should read where there are no competing visual or auditory distractions, and at a time of day when he is most alert. If large text books are available in his topic area, he may find them easier to read. If his periodicals are on-line, printing them out in larger font (e.g., 14–16 point Verdana font) has been found to be preferred by people with aphasia (Worrall, Rose, Howe, McKenna, & Hickson, 2007). He may also choose to intersperse his reading of nonfiction with talking books on the topic. Every attempt would be made to facilitate TC's reading of his preferred texts as it is anticipated that this may improve his reading impairment as well as provide him with topics of conversation so that social participation is enabled. He may also want to consider participating in a book club (Bernstein-Ellis & Elman, 2007), which is often part of UQ groups. Members of the book club read different short sections of the book each week. Each participant provides a brief synopsis of the section they read to the other members so that no one has to read the whole book.

Goal 4: Reading Subtitles

It is expected that reading speed will be the main limiting factor with reading subtexts on foreign films or opera. Two strategies would be discussed with TC. The first is related to priming the words he is about to read by familiarizing himself with the story of the film or opera beforehand. An Internet search might explain the story of the piece while newspapers and the Internet again would provide reviews. The second strategy is similar to the reading strategy of slowly increasing the amount read each day. TC could practice reading subtitles by renting DVDs with subtitles or subscribing to a captioning service for his television. The DVDs would allow him to stop and review the subtext at intervals.

Future group therapy would be used to practice some of the strategies developed in the individual sessions, but most of the group therapy would be targeted at the groups' goals.

Future Sessions

The therapy would continue as above with a large emphasis on collaborative problem solving with TC and rehearsal and practice of skills. Goals are likely to change throughout the block of therapy. It is anticipated that TC's contact with the therapy group, the Association, and the volunteer professor in the Association may provoke some discussions or actions not anticipated earlier. TC may choose to have a large role in the group project, or may become involved in the activities of the Association. New friendships can reduce social isolation that may have developed, although this does not appear to be the case with TC. At the end of the block of therapy, I would review TC's progress. If the goals are still relevant, a repeat of the baseline task as an outcome measure may be appropriate. One final task for all clients (and students and staff) in my client-driven clinic is to review the block of therapy that has taken place by each person describing what they got out of the block of therapy. This qualitative approach often provides a better indicator of outcome than the quantitative baselines and outcomes as the dynamic interaction that has occurred often produces unexpected or immeasurable outcomes. Success of therapy depends on the client meeting his or her own goals or finding some new goals to achieve.

Summary

A client-driven approach with TC has been described. How to use the ICF to conceptualize the rationale for service provision also has been addressed. Interlinking both of these frameworks provides a process whereby the impairment and functional approaches are not mutually exclusive or in competition with each other. In TC's case, a functional or consequences approach was heavily drawn on because his goals were Activity and Participation focused. Impairment-based therapy also is a means to achieve these goals, but it would only be implemented if TC were keen to work intensively on his language. Consequences-focused specialists at UQ also recognize that they probably are not the best service provider in the area of impairment-based language therapy and thus rely heavily on colleagues who specialize in impairment-based therapy. Impairment-based therapy is embraced in the client-driven approach if language goals are important; however, they would not form a large part of therapy for TC because (a) TC's goals are mostly within the Activity/Participation components of the ICF, (b) the client-driven approach views aphasia within a model of disability where both the community and the client need to adjust to living with aphasia, and (c) my own experience shows that positive changes in the broader domains of self-efficacy, participation, and accessibility lead to powerful changes within the community of people with aphasia. Notably, the client-driven approach is only one of several types of service available to people with aphasia at The University of Queensland, so people with aphasia can choose which services they prefer. However, the luxury of choosing the type of service to provide is not always an option in other settings such as public hospitals. However, the client-driven approach could be easily adopted by any speech-language pathologist. This approach does not pit impairment-based approaches against functional approaches. It merely gives much more power to the real specialists in aphasia—the clients with aphasia.

Acknowledgments

The author wishes to acknowledge Dr Tami Howe for her comments on an earlier version of this chapter.

References

Americans with Disability Act of 1990. Available from: http://www.eeoc. gov/policy/ada.html

Basso, A. (2005). How intensive/prolonged should an intensive/prolonged treatment be? *Aphasiology, 19*, 975-984

Bernstein-Ellis, E., & Elman, R. (2007). Aphasia group communication treatment: The Aphasia Center of California Approach. In R. Elman (Ed.), *Group treatment of neurogenic communication disorders: The expert clinician's approach* (2nd ed., pp. 71-94). San Diego, CA: Plural Publishing.

Elman, R. (2007). Introduction to group treatment of neurogenic communication disorders. In R. Elman (Ed.), *Group treatment of neurogenic communication disorders: The expert clinician's approach* (2nd ed., pp. 1-10). San Diego, CA: Plural Publishing.

Elman, R., & Bernstein-Ellis, E. (1999). The efficacy of group communication treatment in adults having chronic aphasia: Linguistic and communication outcome measures. *Journal of Speech, Language and Hearing Research, 42*, 411-419.

Hinckley, J. J., & Packard, M. E. (2001). Family education seminars and social functioning of adults with chronic aphasia. *Journal of Communication Disorders, 34*(3), 241-254.

Hopper, T., Holland, A., & Rewega, M. (2002). Conversational coaching: Treating outcomes and future directions. *Aphasiology, 16*, 745-761.

Kagan, A., Black, S. E., Duchan, J. F., Simmons-Mackie, N., & Square, P. (2001). Training volunteers as conversation partners using "Supported Conversation for Adults with Aphasia" (SCA): A controlled trial. *Journal of Speech, Language and Hearing Research, 44*, 624-638.

Kiresuk, T. J., & Sherman, R. E. (1968). Goal attainment scaling: A general method of evaluating comprehensive community mental health programs. *Community Mental Health Journal, 4*, 443-453.

Lorig, K., Stewart, A., Ritter, P., Gonzalez, V., Laurent, F., & Lynch, J. (1996). *Outcome measures for health education and other health care interventions.* Thousand Oaks, CA: Sage Publications.

Ross, A., Winslow, I., Marchant, P., & Brumfitt, S. (2006). Evaluation of communication, life participation and psychological well-being in chronic aphasia: The influence of group intervention. *Aphasiology, 20*(5), 427-448.

Whitworth, A., Perkins, L., & Lesser, R. (1997). *Conversational Analysis Profile for People with Aphasia (CAPPA).* London: Whurr Publishers.

Worrall, L. (2000). The influence of professional values on the functional communication approach in aphasia. In L. Worrall & C. Frattali (Eds.), *Neurogenic communication disorders: A functional approach.* New York: Thieme.

Worrall, L. E., Davidson, B., Howe, T., & Rose, T. (2007). Clients as teachers: Two aphasia groups at The University of Queensland. In R. Elman (Ed.), *Group treatment of neurogenic communication disorders: The expert clinician's approach* (2nd ed., pp. 137-144). San Diego, CA: Plural Publishing.

Worrall, L., Rose, T., Howe, T., McKenna, K., & Hickson, L. (2007). Developing an evidence-base for accessibility for people with aphasia *Aphasiology, 21*(1), 124-136.

Worrall, L., & Yiu, E. (2000). Effectiveness of functional communication therapy by volunteers for people with aphasia following stroke. *Aphasiology, 14*, 911-924.

13

Impairment and Life Consequences Approaches for Treatment of Nonfluent Aphasia with Agrammatism

Convergences and Divergences

Linda Worrall and Cynthia K. Thompson

There are several ways in which the two approaches to treatment described in this section are compatible. First, both recognize that people with aphasia who are several years postonset of stroke can, and do, improve their language and communication ability, particularly when treatment is provided. Thus, both recommend treatment. The two approaches also embrace the notion that both impairment-based and functionally based approaches are important, and to some extent, components of both are interleaved in their intervention plan. Finally, both approaches use the World Health Organization, International Classification of Functioning, Disability, and Health (WHO-ICF) terminology as a guide for intervention.

There clearly are differences, however, between the two approaches. The impairment-based approach focuses primarily on the presenting deficits of the individual with aphasia and the limitations that they impose for daily communication, whereas, the consequences approach also considers contextual or environmental factors such as communication partners and environments and targets these in intervention. Both interventions recognize that the end goals are functional in nature, but the route to achieve them is different in each case. The impairment-based approach focuses primarily on improving language ability, as noted by improvements on both treated and untreated structures, evaluates the effects of treatment on functional language use, and intervenes to facilitate functional language use when or if it is not forthcoming as a direct result of treatment. Notably, this approach uses stimuli that are relevant to the aphasic person's life, where possible; family members and/or other communication partners are included in treatment planning and evaluation of treatment outcome; and home-practice and group treatment often is included. Treatment begins with a primary focus at the Impairment level, testing, and intervening, if necessary, at the Activity and Participation levels. In contrast, the functional or social model approach focuses intervention primarily at the Activity and Participation levels. The idea is that a change in the Activity or Participation components will have an effect on the Impairment. In addition, changing the environment (a contextual factor) may affect all levels (Impairments, Activity Limitations and Participation Restrictions) experienced by the client. Functional goals at the Activity or Participation level can, therefore, be targeted directly or indirectly by improving surrounding components such as working on the Impairment or the Environment, or a combination of both.

One of the key distinctions between the two approaches pertains to the manner in which treatment targets are chosen. The impairment-based approach is based primarily on the outcome of language testing. The aphasiologist's expertise is required to profile language deficit patterns based on test results, determine the source of the deficit, and design appropriate treatment to address them. The client-driven approach requires that the client is willing and able to participate in decision-making about treatment. The assumption is that the client can indicate their goals and show a preference for treatment options. It also assumes that the client has the expertise to consider and implement strategies to improve their own everyday communication. This does not absolve the therapist from all responsibilities or input into the decision-making process;

both the client and the therapist have specific expertise and responsibilities and the decision-making process, therefore, is collaborative. Depending on the outcome of the decision-making process, treatment may have an impairment focus (bottom-up) or a functional focus (top-down), or both, depending on the client's wishes.

Another difference pertains to the service delivery method. Impairment-based treatment provides one-on-one, client-therapist treatment, and includes group treatment, family member education, and consultation. The functional approach also uses individual and group therapy and consultative and educational components with conversational partners. However, the functional approach requires the therapist to deliver their service in the community (e.g., in adult education classes) as well as in the clinic.

In conclusion, impairment and functional approaches to treatment both aim to improve the communication ability of persons with aphasia. There are several areas in which the two approaches converge, but there also are aspects of the treatments that diverge from one another. Clinicians treating agrammatic aphasia are encouraged to combine the two approaches where possible, to provide optimal opportunities for recovery.

SECTION V

14

A Case of Anomic Aphasia

Nadine Martin and Jacqueline Hinckley

In this section we report on WS, an individual with anomic aphasia and describe two approaches to treating the consequences of his aphasia. One approach focuses on the language impairment specifically, incorporating his personal considerations into his program. The other addresses the state of his overall well-being following the stroke and incorporates language therapy into the program.

Case Description

WS incurred a left-hemisphere stroke when he was 59 years old. A CT scan revealed a lesion involving the inferior frontal, precentral, and anterior superior temporal gyri. The clinical picture at that time included anomic aphasia and a right hemiparesis affecting the upper limb.

WS worked as a lithographer in a printing shop. He completed a 12th grade education and 2 years of technical school. He was working as a printer/lithographer until his stroke occurred. WS has a wide variety of interests including reading, politics, movies, and traveling. He has a close relationship with his wife. He also has a son, who lives at home, and a daughter who lives in another state.

WS is not allowed to drive because of a hemiparesis of the right arm. His wife drives him to therapy and other medical appointments. WS is especially disturbed that his driving is restricted and that he cannot use his arm effectively.

Evaluation of Language Abilities

Despite his anterior lesion and right upper extremity hemiparesis, WS presents with fluent, anomic aphasia. His output is also marked by whole word perseverations. To compensate for his anomia, WS often uses gestures and sound effects (e.g., whistling). He frequently expresses frustration with his inability to retrieve the words he wants to use. Nonetheless, he is pleasant, congenial, and demonstrates a good sense of humor.

Table 14-1 summarizes the results of tests administered to WS to evaluate his receptive and expressive language abilities. These included the Western Aphasia Battery-Revised (WAB-R; Kertesz, 2007), the Pyramids and Palm Trees Test (PPT; Howard & Patter-

Table 14–1. WS: Aphasia Test Scores

Test	Score	Test	Score
Western Aphasia Battery-Revised		**Boston Naming Test**	15/60
Aphasia Quotient	68	**Pyramids and Palm Trees Test**	
Information Content	5/10	Pictures (n = 52)	50/52
Fluency	6/10	Words (n = 52	45/52
Auditory Verbal Comprehension			
Yes/No questions	60/60	**Peabody Picture Vocabulary Test**	
Auditory Word Recognition	60/60	Raw Score	136
Sequential commands	80/80	Standard Score	78
Repetition	82/100		
Naming			
Object Naming	20/100		
Word Fluency	5/20		
Sentence Completion	10/10		
Responsive Speech	8/10		

son, 1992), the Peabody Picture Vocabulary Test (PPVT; Dunn & Dunn, 1981), and the Boston Naming Test (BNT; Kaplan, Goodglass, & Weintraub, 2001),

The results of the WAB were consistent with anomic aphasia. His aphasia quotient was 68. Scores on comprehension subtests were at normal levels and performance on the repetition measures was good. Naming ability was most impaired in the object naming and word fluency subtests, but better performance was noted in sentence completion and responsive speech. This is consistent with the observation that his word retrieval is facilitated easily by phonemic cues and sentence cues, but less so by semantic cues. He attempts to use circumlocutions, but these are usually not informative because the word-retrieval problem is so severe. His performance on the Boston Naming Test (15/60 correct) confirmed a word-retrieval disorder.

As indicated on the WAB, WS's auditory comprehension was generally good, although some mild difficulties appeared in finer measures of comprehension. He had some difficulty with judgments of word associations (45/52) correct on the word version of the PPT test (Howard & Patterson, 1992). Additionally, on the PPVT, a spoken word-to-picture matching test, his score (136) is above the mean (127.54) of a sample of 65 individuals with aphasia, indicating that this ability is only modestly impaired (Martin, Schwartz, & Kohen, 2006).

Communication Goals

WS's expressed goal in therapy is that he be able to say the words he wants to say when he wants to say them.

References

Dunn, L., & Dunn, L. (1981). *Peabody Picture Vocabulary Test-Revised.* Circle Pines, MN: American Guidance Service.

Howard, D., & Patterson, K. (1992). *The Pyramids and Palm Trees test: A test of semantic access from words and pictures.* Bury St. Edmunds, UK: Thames Valley Test Company.

Kaplan, E., Goodglass, H., & Weintraub, S. (2001). *The Boston Naming Test.* (2nd ed). Baltimore: Lippincott, Williams and Wilkins.

Kertesz, A. (2007). *Western Aphasia Battery-Revised.* San Antonio, TX: Harcourt Assessment.

Martin, N., Schwartz, M. F., & Kohen, F. P. (2006). Assessment of the ability to process semantic and phonological aspects of words in aphasia: A multi-measurement approach. *Aphasiology, 20*(2-4), 154–166.

15

Intervention for Anomic Aphasia from a Functional Perspective

Jacqueline Hinckley

Introduction

A functional approach to assessment and intervention has been defined in various ways (Holland & Hinckley, 2002; Worrall, 2000a); however, there are three key concepts that are common across definitions. First, functional approaches prioritize assessment and intervention tools that target communication—both transactional and interactional—within the individual's environment. Thus, a functional approach puts emphasis on individual variation, environmental variation, and their interrelationships. The environment is full of cues that occur in the typical course of events for the individual, and therefore are relevant environmental cues. The individual-environment interaction takes precedence in the clinical process in a functional approach.

Second, a functional approach places emphasis on message content conveyed rather than on message form or communication modality. So, the kind of things that the individual would want to be able to say, and the kinds of communication contexts in which he typically finds himself, will play a primary role in planning assessment and intervention.

There is a third characteristic common across functional approaches. Any variable in the environment is a potential agent for change. In other words, cues and intervention targets are typically sought beyond the boundaries of the clinician-client relationship. A functional approach dictates the consideration of communication partners, communication contexts, environmental adjustments, and the development of internal and/or external strategies to facilitate effective communication.

It has been asserted that an appropriate framework for discussing either a functional approach (Worrall, 2000a) or any theoretical approach to aphasia (Hinckley & Bartels-Tobin, 2007) is the WHO's International Classification of Functioning, Disability, and Health (ICF; WHO, 2001). In a functional approach, contextual variables (or environmental factors) are in the foreground of the clinical problem space. According to the WHO's ICF, environmental factors include products and technologies, changes to the environment, support and relationships, attitudes, and services, systems, and policies. These large categories encompass all aspects of the environment including the intrapersonal, interpersonal, and societal.

In a functional approach to the case of WS, the clinician will first consider typical activities and life participation of the client and how these activities have been affected by the aphasia. Consistent with general principles of a functional approach, the individual's communication arises from the interaction of the individual in his particular context. Contextual information provides a source for goal formulation and prioritization.

Domains from the ICF checklist (WHO, 2003) can be used as a broad rubric for exploring activity limitations and participation restrictions. Is WS limited in his ability to learn and apply knowledge through various formats? Is he limited in his ability to do a single task at one time or his ability to manage multiple tasks? How does his aphasia affect his ability to participate in conversation, or to perform other daily activities such as driving or using transportation, shopping, or meal preparation? Does the aphasia affect his ability to take care of his own health, including understanding medication regimens or making and attending medical appointments? How does his aphasia affect his interpersonal relationships—family, friends, strangers in the community? Is WS able to engage in community life, leisure and recreation pursuits, and civic activities?

Another critical piece of a general functional approach is to assess the environmental facilitators and barriers that will affect WS's activities and life participation. So we would want to know about products and technologies, changes to the environment, support and relationships, attitudes, services, systems, and policies that will either facilitate WS's communication improvement or present a barrier that may need to be overcome. A scan of the environment can provide possible intervention targets or tools that will be important for WS. Finally, the profile of specific cognitive-linguistic abilities and impairments will help to determine which modalities or forms of communication can be used, combined, or supplemented through technology or treatment to achieve the goal of communication in context. Figure 15–1 shows, from a functional perspective, three domains of input to the clinical process for WS. In this view, the profile of cognitive-linguistic impairments is used to help select appropriate treatment procedures, including strategy development.

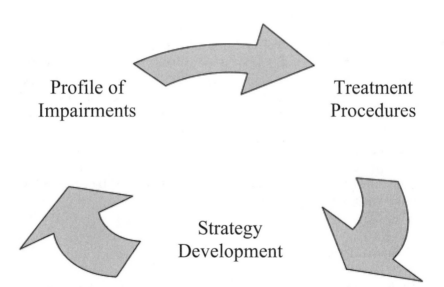

Profile of Impairments

Treatment Procedures

Strategy Development

Figure 15–1. General areas of input to the clinical process for a functional perspective in the case of WS. In this view, the profile of cognitive-linguistic impairments is used to help select appropriate treatment procedures, including strategy development.

Case Interpretation

Review of the available case history and language test data seems to indicate that WS has an anomic aphasia due to a left-hemispheric stroke, without signs of apraxia of speech or dysarthria. Based on the available case information, WS is a lithographer who was literate, socially active, and independent prior to his stroke. He appears to have good social support from his wife and a son who lives nearby, which contributes to a good prognosis for improvement in activities and functions. Using the ICF checklist as a guideline, we can consider various domains of activity and participation, and the following clinical questions arise from incorporating the ICF Checklist to a consideration of the case of WS. We might suspect that WS will have difficulty retaining or learning new verbal information or applying verbal knowledge to daily situations, although we do not have much information about his ability in this area. We also do not know how his performance is affected by distracters in the environment or the need to attend to more than one task at a time. Conversation is significantly affected, based on the case report, and is an area that WS indicates as a priority. With regard to mobility and driving, the case report indicates that his driving limitation is due to his right arm hemiparesis, rather than a language limitation. We do not know about his money management skills for shopping or other home management tasks, nor do we know to what extent WS was previously involved in household tasks, including meal preparation or household duties. We do not know how much assistance he might need with taking medications or other health maintenance tasks. His reading ability has not been assessed and so we do not know specifically how his leisure pursuit of reading might potentially be affected by his aphasia except by his self-report of difficulty with newspaper items.

Additional Assessment

The ICF framework helps to point out areas in which additional information is required to plan an effective intervention program. First, more information about what WS considers to be important communication activities and life goals is needed—at this point we only know that he wants to improve his ability to say the words he wants to say. What daily activities or life goals does he want to accomplish? We can assess this more fully with the use of an extended interview (Lyon & Shadden, 2001; Simmons-Mackie, 2001). Another interesting approach to eliciting information about participation in life activities is the use of a picture card sort (Haley et al., 2005). Similarly, it will be important to interview his wife to gain her perspective on the impact of WS's aphasia on the performance of household activities, the pursuit of leisure activities, and the dynamics of their own relationship and relationships with other family members and friends (Pound, Parr, & Duchan, 2001; Sorin-Peters, 2004).

Part of the interview can be used to determine how WS previously spent his time and to prioritize these activities in terms of time management and value to the client (Lyon & Shadden, 2001; Simmons-Mackie, 2001). This can be compared to a description of how WS currently uses his time and what activities he currently engages in. This will help to determine intervention priorities. Repeating such an assessment after an intervention can also help to determine whether the intervention made any impact on WS's life participation.

A possible guide to the interviewing process might be the completion of a measure such as the Community Integration Questionnaire (Willer, Rosenthal, Kreutzer, Gordon, & Rempel, 1993). This structured interview tool provides opportunities to respond to questions about household chores, visits outside the home, and participation in volunteer/work activities. It is a relatively short measure that could be readministered at the end of an intervention period to measure potential life participation outcomes at the level of household and community involvement.

Given the extent of WS's anomia and his own indication that saying what he wants to say is a priority, further assessment of conversational breakdowns that will lead to development of effective conversational strategies will be necessary. Conversational samples should be gathered at least with WS interacting with an unfamiliar partner and with his wife. Quantitative analysis of content and informational units, such as Correct Information Unit analysis (Nicholas & Brookshire, 1993) may be appropriate as a measure associated with his naming abilities. Perhaps more importantly, though, a qualitative conversational analysis should be used to describe the nature of communication breakdowns between WS and his partner, and what techniques both WS and his partner use to repair these break-downs (Damico & Oelschlager, 1999; Oelschlaeger & Damico, 1998, 1999; Prins & Baastianse, 2004). It may be that repair strategies used by WS differ in his interactions with his wife versus unfamiliar partners. It will also be of utmost importance to analyze the communication strategies used by his wife and assess them for effectiveness.

The Communicative Abilities in Daily Living assessment (CADL-2; Holland, Frattali, & Fromm, 1999) would be an appropriate tool to help assess the client's strengths and weaknesses for activities like shopping, reading prescriptions, and attending medical appointments. An alternative assessment here could be the Amersterdam-Nijmegen Everyday Language Test (ANELT; Blomert, Kean, & Koster, 1994). His performance on a test like this might point out areas of daily activities that are being affected by the aphasia, and provide an opportunity for discussion between the clinician, WS, and his wife about the relative importance of those activities in the life of WS

Additional structured assessments are also indicated to help identify an appropriate course of intervention. These additional structured assessments should be selected based on the activity and life participation priorities arrived at through interviewing techniques with WS and his wife. WS indicated, as mentioned in the case report, that he was having some difficulty reading newspaper items. As reading has been indicated as one of WS's hobbies, it may deserve further assessment attention. Reading assessments that measure silent reading comprehension at the paragraph level or lengthier material would be appropriate to pursue the identification of treatment goals and strategies for reading (e.g., Brookshire & Nicholas, 1997; LaPointe & Horner, 1998). Any reading assessment should focus on the potential compensatory strategies that aid his reading success.

We also do not know anything about WS's writing abilities from the case report, and this might be an important area to assess as it might serve as an effective communication means in certain contexts. Can he retrieve the first letter of target words? If so, can he use any preserved grapheme-to-phoneme correspondence ability to self-cue? Can he use writing for social involvement or the completion of daily activities (Parr, 1992, 1995)?

Because a functional approach to intervention implies the potential use of a variety of communication strategies, it is important to know the strengths and limitations of WS's cognitive abilities, such as executive function (Purdy, 2006; Ramsberger, 2005). This is likely to help the clinician predict the complexity level of strategies that will be appropriate for WS, how much training and what kind of training might be most beneficial, and whether WS is likely to be able to generalize or transfer a strategy learned in one context to a different context. The Cognitive-Linguistic Quick Test (Helm-Estabrooks, 2001) is an example of a cognitive screening tool that was designed for use with adults with aphasia. Subtests assess attention, memory, visual-spatial skills, and executive function (as well as language) through the use of stimulus materials that are nonlinguistic in nature. An alternative cognitive assessment to consider is the Global Aphasia Neuropsychological Battery (van Mourik, Verschaeve, Boon, Paquier, & van Harskamp, 1992). This composite of assessments targeting attention, memory, visual-spatial abilities, and reasoning were originally designed for use with adults with severe aphasia. However, it can be used with clients with a broad range of aphasia severities (Hinckley & Nash, in press; Hinckley, Patterson, & Carr, 2001).

Finally, we do not yet know how WS's language performance is affected by distraction or the performance of multiple tasks at once. Again, assessments in this area would be indicated only if WS tends to be in a distracting or busy environment, or if he plans to be in such environments. There are few well-developed clinical assessment measures in this area (for a review see Murray, 1999). Although there are tasks that have been used for research purposes and might be adapted for clinical uses, these tasks would serve as a criterion-based assessment only. For example, Murray (2004) investigated the effects of varying attentional demands on single-word retrieval abilities in addition to exploring the effects of a tone detection task on picture description abilities (Murray, Holland, & Beeson, 1998). McNeil et al. (2004) similarly used story retell and tracking tasks. An ecologically useful task—ordering items from a catalog—was administered to adults with aphasia in a dual-task paradigm with a tone detection component (Hinckley, Carr & Patterson, submitted for publication; Hinckley, Patterson, & Carr, 2001). These tasks reveal the sensitivity of communication abilities to distraction and cognitive load, are sensitive to changes in relation to treatment, and can demonstrate increased robustness of communication abilities as a result of training.

Treatment Goals

With the preeminence of the interrelationships between the individual and context in a functional approach comes a corresponding collaborative tone to the client-clinician relationship. Worrall (2000b) describes a model of shared decision-making between client and clinician, in which power within the therapeutic relationship is shared. In this model, both clinician and client have information to share with the other, and consensus about the preferred treatment approach is achieved through multilateral discussions. Such a model acknowledges the emphasis on individual differences that is inherent in the functional approach. Development of treatment goals would need, therefore, to be achieved jointly and collaboratively with the client and his wife, so that they are built upon their priorities, tempered by the knowledge and experience of the clinician. Furthermore, the intervention time available and environmental factors that serve as facilitators or barriers should drive additional treatment goal selection.

Given that such a process has been completed, the following goals seem appropriate for WS.

1. Improve conversational success between WS and his wife so that successful exchanges increase and breakdowns are repaired successfully.
2. Improve conversational abilities with friends or others in the community.
3. Facilitate development of successful reading strategies so that WS can enjoy reading the newspaper or other items for pleasure.
4. Ensure that WS can use appropriate money skills for the completion of daily activities such as shopping.
5. Facilitate language skills required for passing a driving exam, if indicated.
6. Improve ability to achieve communicative/conversational success in distracting environments such as restaurants or with the TV on in the background.

Treatment(s)

From the functional perspective, the nature of the anomic episodes within the social context is the primary point of intervention. When the client has word retrieval difficulty within a conversation, what happens? What does he do, and what does his partner do? How can effective communication take place, regardless of modality or strategy?

Based on the conversational analysis, strategies that are successful for WS and his wife and the circumstances under which they are beneficial can be identified. Then, based on the set of preserved communication skills and abilities that the two of them together possess, a menu of conversational strategies can be developed and agreed on in rank order of usefulness.

One organized approach to developing effective strategies for an individual with aphasia and his or her partner is Conversational Coaching (Hopper, Holland, & Rewega, 2002). For example, if WS's wife is unsure of his intended meaning in conversation, perhaps she could ask WS to provide more information. He may then be able to use circumlocution as a useful conversational strategy by providing additional information that allows his partner to construct the intended meaning with him. Another alternative might be to write the first letter or other graphical information about a key word in the conversation. Depending on how useful the identified strategies are, which ones are most effective, and which ones are preferred by WS and his wife, a menu of conversational strategies can be developed and agreed on in rank order of usefulness. These strategies are developed with the help of the clinician and tested in somewhat controlled situations. The Conversational Coaching technique typically involves the use of short videotaped examples that are watched by one person (either WS or his wife) and the two take turns working together, using their conversational strategies to share the story in the videotaped segment.

Because we do not know about WS's writing abilities, we can not guess as to whether writing might play a role in his effective conversational strategy repertoire (e.g., Dede, Parris, & Waters, 2003). The case report does suggest that circumlocution occasionally works to facilitate word retrieval, and this might be an area for the development of a specific strategy (e.g., Francis, Clark, & Humphreys, 2002). .

It will be important to enter into the treatment selection equation the results of the cognitive assessment, particularly in regard to executive function. Some evidence suggests that executive function as measured by clinical assessments is linked to the ability to identify, retrieve, and deploy communication strategies during a conversation (Purdy, 2006). Executive function may also be critical to the ability to shift from one communication strategy to another (e.g., from using circumlocution to writing single letters or partial words) while maintaining conversational goals and topics.

The potential relationship between executive function and treatment parameters such as practice context and number of repetitions should also be considered. Individuals with lower executive function may be less able to identify cues in the environment that should trigger certain communication responses, such as the implementation of a conversational strategy. For these individuals, practice should occur in a context that shares the maximum number of characteristics with the target context where implementation is hoped for. When practice within therapy shares important contextual cues such as conversational partner (WS's wife) and likely conversational topics, then the likelihood that WS. will use these same strategies outside of therapy is increased.

If intervention beginning at the conversational level appears to be ineffective for WS, then the conversational skill targeted could be decomposed from the larger task and practiced separately, then reintegrated into the target context of conversation. In the case of WS., perhaps the use of circumlocution as a conversational strategy is initially too challenging, even though he is able to produce circumlocution in a basic picture-naming task. It might follow that an improved ability to use circumlocution in a "simpler" task, like picture naming, might increase his ease or fluency in producing circumlocution. As this ease with the specific skill increases, his ability to use this as an effective communication strategy in conversation might also increase, and the "decomposed" skill of circumlocution can be reintroduced into a conversational setting. This follows from the literature suggesting that part-task training is generally more effective for complex tasks (Donovan & Radesovich, 1999). But in the typical approach to part-task training, decomposable skills are always practiced again in the context of the larger task after mastery in the decomposed condition. Practice in a context that shares a number of cues to the target environment is critical, because those contextual cues will serve as the retrieval cue for implementation of the conversational strategy.

.With regard to communication with unfamiliar partners, WS may benefit from script training (Youmans, Holland, & Munoz,

2005). Script training involves the identification of a personalized script or dialogue that is overpracticed and then can be used in various social settings. Many people are familiar with memorizing dialogues during foreign language learning, and script training has many elements in common with this type of specific language form learning. For example, an individual with aphasia might wish to learn a "script" that explains why they have trouble communicating and what others can do to communicate effectively with him or her. The desired message is written out with the help of the clinician and agreed on. Massed practice of the script is accomplished alone and also with a variety of communication partners. Ultimately, the script becomes overlearned and rehearsed and can be relatively easily retrieved in any context.

Script training is likely to be effective for WS because of his responsiveness to phonemic cuing, with the potential interpretation that overpractice of the phonological forms of words, particularly words that are important to him and tell something about him as a person, could lead to improved use of those particular words. An additional potential benefit of script training is that overpracticed word forms in a script might generalize to production of those words in other contexts, even when the script itself is not being produced.

Outcome Measures

Direct effects of the treatment should be measured as the primary outcomes. Indirect effects should also be measured as a way to determine how much transfer and generalization, if any, has occurred. This can also help to determine whether additional treatment would be beneficial, and if so, what the target or nature of that treatment should be.

Direct effects of the conversational treatment that should be measured are the ability of WS and his wife to communicate messages effectively. Content units in discourse should be measured and compared to the pretreatment abilities. Conversational effectiveness between WS and his wife can be measured by the number of turns required to communicate a message, and the relative proportion of successfully implemented repairs of conversational breakdowns.

Similarly, WS's ability to convey basic information about himself or a given message to unfamiliar communication partners should also be measured as a direct effect of the script-based training. The number of correct and meaningful words and ideas conveyed to an unfamiliar partner would be a meaningful measure of the potential effects of this treatment.

Outcome measures from each of the ICF levels—impairment, activity, and participation—should also be taken to determine whether this particular treatment regimen produced other effects besides those that seemed to be directly linked to the treatment. In the case of WS, a life activities inventory to determine whether he has changed the relative amount of time spent in various activities, or most especially, activities that are desirable to him, would be an important measure to determine whether this treatment was sufficient to impact life participation or whether a more direct intervention focused on those specific activities is warranted. This measure would most likely be more telling than a generic measure of community integration, like the *Community Integration Questionnaire* (CIQ) (Willer et al., 1993) or even a more generic measure of perceived quality of life. It could be argued that assessing WS's participation in activities that he deemed to be most personally relevant and important is a type of individual-specific quality of life measure.

It will be critical to obtain the viewpoint of others in WS's environment, most especially his wife, as to whether change has occurred with regard to WS's communication abilities. The Communicative Effectiveness Index (CETI; Lomas et al., 1989) is a reliable measure for obtaining the perceptions of others regarding communication change. The communication partner—in this case, WS's wife—is asked to rate WS's ability to perform a number of specified communication activities on a visual analog scale. When this is completed both before and after a course of therapy, perceived relative change can be reliably assessed.

Depending on the results of the additional assessments administered prior to initiation of treatment, it may be useful to readminister a measure associated with the activity level. Administration of the CADL-2 (Holland, Frattali, & Fromm, 1999) would provide an opportunity to assess whether improvement in the use of conversational strategies were generalized to use in other contexts, such as the shopping and medical appointment contexts role-played during this test.

Finally, an impairment-level measure should also be administered to determine whether conversational-level treatment produced transfer to naming improvement on traditional picture-naming measures. Thus, the picture-naming assessments, such as the Philadelphia Naming Test (Roach, Schwartz, Martin, Grewal, & Brecher, 1996), that were administered prior to treatment initiation should be readministered. Conversation requires the deployment of a variety of cognitive and linguistic abilities; thus, it is reasonable to at least explore the possibility that "higher level" treatment such as conversational treatment might transfer to "lower-level" skills such as "simple naming" in a picture-naming test.

There is reason to suspect that such a transfer might well occur. First, a number of studies have recently demonstrated an effect in which training on more complex members of a category or domain generalize to improvement on untrained simpler category members. This has been termed the Complexity Account of Treatment Efficacy (Thompson, 2007; Thompson, Shapiro, Kiran, & Sobecks, 2003). The Complexity Effect has been observed in aphasia in semantic (Kiran, 2007; Stanczak, Waters, & Caplan, 2006) and syntactic (Thompson, Shapiro, Kiran, & Sobecks, 2003) domains. It is conceptually feasible that the general principle could be observed in generalization from complex contexts like conversation to less complex or "decontextualized" measures at the impairment level.

Another argument for the potential generalization from contextually rich training environments to less contextualized performance environments follows from theoretical models derived from connectionist approaches. The richer the training context, the more contextual cues are available to serve as retrieval cues for later performance (e.g., MacWhinney, 1987). A relationship between a contextually rich training environment and generalization to improvement on a decontextualized measure, specifically picture naming, was observed in the work of Hinckley, Carr, and Patterson (2001).

Certainly, impairment-oriented treatments typically measure performance in higher order communication tasks like conversation, with the hope that the impairment-based treatment will have generalized, often without specific conversational training, to that desirable context. Functional approaches to communication should likewise measure potential effects on impairments so that we might further understand the complex relations between what we perceive as transferable skills, like picture naming, to more global and highly contextualized communication performances, such as conversation.

Summary

This description of a functional approach to WS's treatment illustrates four important points.

1. Activities and life participation that are relevant and important for the individual are used to drive assessment decisions and to prioritize treatment goals.
2. Any contextual factor has an equal potential to serve as an agent of change in the functional perspective—physical environmental factors, conversational partners, attitudes and beliefs, remediation of a specific impairment.
3. The profile of cognitive-linguistic impairments contributes to the selection and development of appropriate treatment strategies, procedures, and treatment type (including treatment contexts, rate, and duration of practice).
4. Outcomes should be measured at all levels—impairment, activity, and participation—because we do not know yet to what extent manipulation of any given environmental factor might affect impairment, activity, or participation.

References

Blomert, L., Kean, M.-L., & Koster, C. (1994). Amsterdam-Nijmegen Everyday Language Test: Construction, reliability and validity. *Aphasiology, 8,* 381–407.

Brookshire, R., & Nicholas, L. E. (1997). *Discourse Comprehension Test.* Minneapolis, MN: BRK Publishers.

Damico, J. S., & Oelschlaeger, M. (1999). Qualitative methods in aphasia research: Conversation analysis. *Aphasiology, 13,* 667–679.

Dede, G., Parris, D., & Waters, G. (2003). Teaching self-cues: A treatment approach for verbal naming. *Aphasiology, 17,* 465–480.

Donovan, J. J., & Radosevich, D. J. (1999). A meta-analytic review of the distribution of practice effect: Now you see it, now you don't. *Journal of Applied Psychology, 84,* 795–805.

Francis, D. R., Clark, N., & Humphreys, G. W. (2002). Circumlocution-induced naming (CIN): A treatment for effecting generalization in anomia? *Aphasiology, 16,* 243–259.

Haley, K., Jenkins, K., Hadden, C., Womack, J. Hall, J., & Schwiker, C. (2005). Sorting pictures to assess participation in life activities. *Perspectives on Neurophysiology and Neurogenic Speech and Language Disorders, 15*(4), 11–15.

Helm-Estabrooks, N. (2001). *Cognitive Linguistic Quick Test.* San Antonio, TX: The Psychological Corporation.

Hinckley, J. J., & Bartels-Tobin, L. (2007). Assessment of aphasia. In A. F. Johnson & B. H. Jacobson (Eds.), *Medical speech-language pathology: A practitioner's guide* (2nd ed.). New York: Thieme.

Hinckley, J. J., Carr, T. H., & Patterson, J. P. (submitted for publication). Development of a multi-tasking functional assessment for aphasia. *Aphasiology.*

Hinckley, J. J. & Nash, C. (in press). Cognitive assessment and aphasia severity. *Brain and Language.*

Hinckley, J. J., Patterson, J., & Carr, T. H. (2001). Differential effects of context- and skill-based treatment approaches: Preliminary findings. *Aphasiology, 15,* 463–476.

Holland, A., Frattali, C., & Fromm, D. (1999). *Communication Activities of Daily Living* (2nd ed.). Austin, TX: Pro-Ed.

Holland, A. L., & Hinckley, J. J. (2002). Assessment and treatment of pragmatic aspects of communication in aphasia. In A. Hillis (Ed.), *Handbook on adult language disorders: Integrating cognitive neuropsychololgy, neurology and rehabilitation.* Philadelphia: Psychology Press.

Hopper, T. Holland, A., & Rewega, M. (2002). Conversational coaching: Treatment outcomes and future directions. *Aphasiology, 16,* 745–761.

ICF. (2001). *International Classification of Functioning, Disability, and Health*: ICF. Geneva: World Health Organization.

Kiran, S. (2007). Complexity in the treatment of naming deficits. *American Journal of Speech-Language Pathology, 16,* 18–29.

LaPointe, L. L., & Horner, J. (1998). *Reading Comprehension Battery for Aphasia* (2nd ed.). New York: Harcourt Brace.

Lomas, J.. Pickard, L., Bester, S., Elbard, H., Finlayson, A., & Zochaib, C. (1989). The Communicative Effectiveness Index: Development and psychometric evaluation of a functional communication measure for adult aphasia. *Journal of Speech and Hearing Disorders, 54,* 113–124.

Lyon, J. G., & Shadden, B. B. (2001). Treating life consequences of aphasia's chronicity. In R. Chapey (Ed.), *Language intervention strategies in aphasia and related neurogenic communication disorders.* Philadelphia: Lippincott Williams & Wilkins,

MacWhinney, B. (1987). The competition model. In B. MacWhinney (Ed.), *Mechanisms of language acquisition* (pp. 249–308). Hillsdale, NJ: Erlbaum.

McNeil, M. R., Doyle, P. J., Hula, W. D., Rubinsky, H. R., Fossett, T. R. D., & Matthews, C. T. (2004). Using resource allocation theory and dual-task methods to increase the sensitivity of assessment in aphasia. *Aphasiology, 18,* 521–542.

Murray, L. L. (1999). Attention and aphasia: Theory, research, and clinical implications. *Aphasiology, 13,* 91–111.

Murray, L. L. (2004). Cognitive treatments for aphasia: Should we and can we help attention and working memory problems? *Medical Journal of Speech-Language Pathology, 12,* xxi–xxxviii.

Murray, L. L., Holland, A. L., & Beeson, P. M. (1998). Spoken language of individuals with mild fluent aphasia under focused and divided attention conditions. *Journal of Speech, Language, and Hearing Research, 41,* 213–227.

Nicholas, L., & Brookshire, R. (1993). A system for quantifying the informativeness and efficiency of connected speech in adults with aphasia. *Journal of Speech and Hearing Research, 36,* 338–350.

Oelschlaeger, M., & Damico, J. (1998). Spontaneous verbal repetition: A social strategy in aphasic conversation. *Aphasiology, 12,* 971–988.

Oelschlaeger, M., & Damico, J. (1999). Participation of a conversation partner in the word searches of a person with aphasia. *American Journal of Speech-Language Pathology, 8,* 62–71.

Parr, S. (1992). Everyday reading and writing practices of normal adults: Implications for aphasia assessment. *Aphasiology, 6,* 273–283.

Parr, S. (1995). Everyday reading and writing in aphasia: Role change and the influence of pre-morbid literacy practice. *Aphasiology, 9,* 223–238.

Pound, C., Parr, S., & Duchan, J. (2001). Using partners' autobiographical reports to develop, deliver and evaluate services in aphasia. *Aphasiology, 15,* 477–493.

Prins, R., & Baastianse, R. (2004). Analyzing the spontaneous speech of aphasic speakers. *Aphasiology, 18,* 1075–1091.

Purdy, M. (2006). Prediction of strategy usage by adults with aphasia. *Aphasiology, 20,* 337–348.

Ramsberger, G. (2005). Achieving conversational success in aphasia by focusing on non-linguistic cognitive skills: A potentially promising new approach. *Aphasiology, 19,* 1066–1073.

Roach, A., Schwartz, M. F., Martin, N., Grewal, R. S., & Brecher, A. (1996). The Philadelphia Naming Test: Scoring and rationale. *Clinical Aphasiology, 24,* 121–133.

Simmons-Mackie, N. (2001). Social approaches to aphasia intervention. In Chapey, R. (Ed.), *Language intervention strategies in aphasia and related neurogenic communication disorders* (pp. 246–266). Philadelphia: Lippincott Williams & Wilkins.

Sorin-Peters, R. (2004). The evaluation of a learner-centred training programme for spouses of adults with chronic aphasia using qualitative case study methodology. *Aphasiology, 18*, 951-975.

Stanczak, L., Waters, G., & Caplan, D. (2006). Typicality-based learning and generalisation in aphasia: Two case studies of anomia treatment. *Aphasiology, 20*, 374-383.

Thompson, C. K. (2007). Complexity in language learning and treatment. *American Journal of Speech-Language Pathology, 16*, 3-5.

Thompson, C. K., Shapiro, L. P., Kiran, S., & Sobecks, J. (2003). The role of syntactic complexity in treatment of sentence deficits in agrammatic aphasia: The complexity account of treatment efficacy (CATE). *Journal of Speech, Language, and Hearing Research, 46*, 591-607.

van Mourik, M., Verschaeve, M., Boon, P., Paquier, P., & van Harskamp, F. (1992). Cognition in global aphasia: Indicators for therapy. *Aphasiology, 6*, 491-499.

Willer, B., Rosenthal, M., Kreutzer, J. S., Gordon, W. A., & Rempel, R. A. (1993). Assessment of community integration following traumatic brain injury. *Journal of Head Trauma Rehabilitation, 8*, 75-87.

World Health Organization. (2003). *ICF checklist.* Geneva: World Health Organization.

Worrall, L. E. (2000a). A conceptual framework for a functional approach to acquired neurogenic disorders of communication and swallowing. In L. E. Worrall & C. M. Frattal (Eds.), *Neurogenic communication disorders: A functional approach* (pp. 3-18). New York: Thieme.

Worrall, L. E. (2000b). The influence of professional values on the functional communication approach in aphasia. In L. E. Worrall & C. M. Frattali (Eds.), *Neurogenic communication disorders: A functional approach.* (pp. 191-205). New York: Thieme.

Youmans, G.. Holland, A., & Munoz, M. (2005). Script training and automaticity n two individuals with aphasia. *Aphasiology, 19*, 435-450.

16

Intervention for Anomic Aphasia from a Cognitive Impairment-Based Perspective

Nadine Martin

Case Interpretation

The primary goal of language testing is to establish a language ability profile in the context of a model of language processing. This process coupled with treatments that are tailor made to treat a particular type of language deficit has been termed "hypothesis' testing" (e.g., Caplan, 1993; Gagnon & Martin, 2002, Raymer & Gonzalez Rothi, 2002). Each test result provides clues that lead to an hypothesis of the locus/loci of breakdown in language processing that is present. The test of that hypothesis is observed via the efficacy of a treatment designed to target that particular deficit.

Results of administration of the WAB, the BNT, and the PPVT indicate a language profile consistent with anomic aphasia. Speech output is fluent (fluency score of 6/10) and naming is severely impaired (score 20/100). In contrast, auditory comprehension and repetition are relatively spared, although mild impairments in both domains are evident. Clearly, assessment of WS's language ability reveals a profound difficulty retrieving words. His performance on the picture and word versions of the PPT (Howard & Patterson, 1992) is informative with respect to the source of his anomia. This test examines the integrity of the semantic system and access to that system from words in a task that involves judging associations of concepts represented in pictures or in words. His good performance on the picture version (52/52) indicates that his naming deficit is likely not due to an impairment of semantic knowledge. However, his score on the verbal version (46/52) indicates some possible difficulties in accessing the semantic system from words. In production, a disturbance of the connections between semantics and phonological forms of words may be the source of his word retrieval deficit. Producing a word involves several stages that reflect semantic, lexical, or phonological processing. In order to develop an accurate language profile, it is important to examine all aspects of word retrieval in sufficient detail to determine the locus of the breakdown. This was accomplished through additional testing described in the next section.

Additional Assessment

The model shown in Figure 16–1 is typical of functional models of word processing, which provide a useful framework within which to evaluate word processing ability. The case interpretation helps to identify which stages of the word retrieval process are impaired and provides some insight into the nature of the impairment. The importance of gaining a complete profile of language abilities and deficits cannot be underestimated. This profile will enable the clinician to design tasks that stimulate semantic or phonological processing abilities or both (Laine & Martin, 2006).

The following tests were administered (Table 16–1) to help clarify the locus of WS's impairment: the Philadelphia Comprehension Battery (PCB; Saffran, Schwartz, Linebarger, Martin, & Bochetto, 1987), the Philadelphia Naming Test (PNT; Roach, Schwartz, Martin, Grewal, & Brecher, 1996), portions of the Psycholinguistic Assessments of Language Processing in Aphasia (PALPA; Kay, Lesser, & Coltheart 1992), and measurements of digit and word span (Martin & Ayala, 2002).

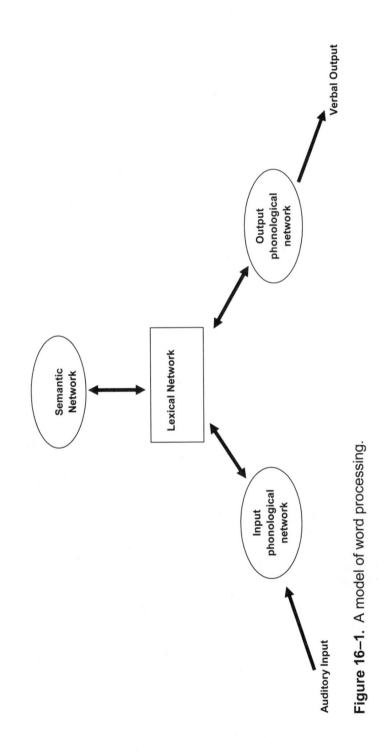

Figure 16–1. A model of word processing.

Table 16–1. WS: Results of Additional testing Test

Test	Score	Test	Score
Philadelphia Naming Test	49/175	Psycholinguistic Assessments of Language Processing in Aphasia (PALPA) (continued)	
Philadelphia Comprehension Battery			
Word-to-picture matching		*Word Repetition PALPA 7*	
Within category distractors	14/16	1 syllable	7/8
Across category distractors	16/16	2 syllable	7/8
Synonymy Judgments		3 syllable	5/8
Nouns	11/15	*Nonword Repetition PALPA 8*	
Verbs	9/15	1 syllable	6/8
Sentence Comprehension		2 syllable	6/8
Reversible semantic roles	53/60	3 syllable	4/8
Nonreversible semantic roles	57/60	*Word Repetition: Imageability and Frequency PALPA 9*	
Grammaticality Judgments		High Imageability	39/40
Recognize correct sentences	28/30	Low imageability	33/40
		High Frequency	38/40
Recognize incorrect sentences	14/30	Low Frequency	34/40
Psycholinguistic Assessments of Language Processing in Aphasia (PALPA)		*Grammatical Class Reading PALPA 32*	
		Nouns	12/20
		Adjectives	10/20
		Verbs	9/20
Same-Different Discrimination (nonwords) PALPA 1		Functors	4/20
		Auditory Short-Term Memory	
Same	34/36	*Repetition Span*	
Different	35/36	Digits	3
Same-Different Discrimination (words) PALPA 2		Words	2
		Pointing Span	
Same	35/36	Digits	2
Different	35/36	Words	3

continues

Table 16–1. *(continued)*

Test	Score	Test	Score
Auditory Lexical Decision: Imageabilty and Frequency PALPA 5			
High Imageability	37/40		
Low imageability	34/40		
High Frequency	36/40		
Low Frequency	35/40		

Picture Naming and Word Retrieval

A good place to begin supplementary testing is to examine WS's picture-naming ability in greater detail. The low scores on the WAB naming and BNT indicated impaired word retrieval; however, further testing is needed to tease out the locus of his naming deficit. We start with administration of the PNT (Roach et al., 1996), a 175-item picture naming test developed by researchers at Temple University and Moss Rehabilitation Research Institute. Normative data on this test are available in Roach et al. (1996), and the test itself is available from the authors. Consistent with results on the WAB and the BNT, WS demonstrated severe naming difficulty on this test (score 28% correct naming). In-depth evaluation of the types of errors he made provides further clues about the locus of disruption. Many "no response" errors as well as omissions, whole word perseverations, and semantic errors were noted. His typical response to a picture he could not name was "I know it, but I can't say it." Whole word perseverations indicated an inability to overcome persistent activation of previous utterances and suggested a breakdown in processes that enable the conceptual-semantic system to access the word form and phonology of an intended utterance. The fact that WS produced few if any phonological errors in naming suggests that connections between the lexical-phonological form of a word and the phonemes of that word (the phonological encoding stage) are intact. This suggestion is supported by his good performance on the WAB repetition subtests, but further testing of lexical-semantic, syntactic, and phonological processing, as well as verbal short-term memory (STM) is needed to confirm this hypothesis.

Further Tests of Lexical-Semantic
Abilities and Sentence Comprehension

What is the nature of the deficit that is inhibiting access to the word form from semantics? WS's performance on tests of semantic processing indicates a mild impairment in this domain that appears to affect access to semantic representations rather than impaired semantic knowledge. Evidence for this includes variability in word retrieval success, depending on task characteristics (complexity and working memory requirements) and demonstration of semantic knowledge on nonverbal tests (PPT; Howard & Patterson, 1992). To further examine lexical-semantic and sentence processing, WS was administered the Philadelphia Comprehension Battery (PCB; Saffran et al., 1987). This test has four subtests, two of which examine access to lexical-semantic information and two of which examine comprehension of sentences. His performance on the sentence comprehension subtest of the PCB indicates mild difficulty comprehending sentences with reversible semantic roles. There is also some evidence on the grammaticality judgments subtest of difficulty in recognizing grammatical errors in sentences.

The tests of lexical-semantic processing in this battery reveal more insight into his word retrieval disorder. The Lexical Comprehension subtest is a spoken word-to-picture matching task that uses the same format as the PPVT (Dunn & Dunn, 1981). A word is spoken and the participant's task is to choose one of four pictures that match the spoken word. Spoken word-to-picture matching tasks can reveal important information about lexical-semantic impairments by varying the relationship between the distractor items and the target item. The Lexical Comprehension subtest compares performance on a condition in which distractors are semantically related to the target (e.g., target: *carrot*, distractors: celery, peas, onion) with one that has unrelated distractors (e.g., target: *carrot*, distractors: horse, hammer, shirt). Better performance on the condition with unrelated distractors has been interpreted as evidence for underspecified semantic representations (Hillis, 1991), indicating that the person has knowledge of the general category of a word (carrot is a vegetable) but cannot differentiate it from other vegetables. More recent interpretations regard this pattern as evidence for an access problem. Activation of related items in the lexicon causes competition among these items and can result in interference. This has been referred to as a refractory access problem (Crutch & Warrington, 2005).

WS's performance is mildly impaired on spoken word-to-picture matching tasks when the items to choose from are semantically related. When the pictures to choose from share no relationship, his performance is at ceiling. This performance pattern suggests instability in accessing semantic concepts from spoken words.

Additional evidence of an impairment in accessing semantics from words comes from WS's performance on the Synonymy Judgment subtest of the PCB. This test involves judging the similarity of meanings of two or more words. Any comparison task engages short-term working memory to some degree; however, STM demands can vary, depending on the paradigm used. The synonymy tasks used in WS's evaluation involved listening to three spoken words and simultaneously viewing their written forms (e.g., jail, prison, cage). He was then asked to think about what each word means and determine which two are most similar in meaning (jail, prison). WS performed poorly on this task and made more errors judging verb meanings (9/15 correct) than noun meanings (11/15 correct). Thus, he demonstrated greater difficulty on this lexical-semantic task that requires accessing and *maintaining activation* of word meanings in short-term memory.

In another version of this paradigm, the participant is presented with one word (e.g., jail) and then presented with two more words (prison, cage). The task is used to determine which of the latter two words is most similar in meaning to the first word presented. In terms of working memory load, this task requires maintaining only two pairs of words in STM. Performance on synonymy judgments using this paradigm has been shown to improve performance compared to the three-pair version (Kohen, Kalinyak-Fliszar, & Martin, 2006), even after differences in chance levels of performance are considered. Although the two-pair version of the task was not administered to WS, he was tested on the PPT (Howard & Patterson, 1992), which does use this format for an association judgment task. In that test, a word or a picture is presented (e.g., pyramid) and then two words or two pictures (palm tree, pine tree) are presented and the participant decides which of those two is most associated with the first picture or word. As noted in the case description, WS's score on the word version of the PPT test (46/52) was lower than his score on the picture version (52/52), but just below the normal range.

If a semantic knowledge deficit is present, performance on all of these judgment tasks would be similar regardless of the format used. If the difficulty is one of accessing and maintaining activation of verbal input and associated semantic representations, performance would vary depending on two factors: the verbal content (word class, imageability, similarity with other words being processed in the task), and task demands, particularly the degree to which the task stresses STM working capacity. WS had more difficulty with judgment tasks that put a greater load on short-term working memory (i.e., synonymy judgments for nouns and verbs). He also showed word class effects, being better able to judge meanings of nouns compared to verbs and concrete words compared to abstract words.

Evaluation of Input and Output Lexical-Phonological Processing

The PALPA was administered to gain insight into WS's phonological processing abilities and his sensitivity to language variables that affect comprehension, repetition and reading of words such as phonological similarity, imageability of words, syllable length, and word class. As Table 16–1 indicates, his performance on these subtests indicated intact phoneme discrimination abilities, good word recognition (no strong effect of imageability), and adequate ability to repeat single words with only mild effects of syllable length, frequency, and imageability. Oral reading of content words was good, although there were effects of word class (difficulty reading functor words). Reading comprehension was not formally assessed, although WS reported that he had some difficulty understanding text in newspapers.

Assessment of Verbal Short-Term Memory Abilities

Thus far, the interpretation of WS's language evaluation has focused on the impaired aspects of his language ability. These involve mostly lexical and semantic processing of words. WS's ability to process phonological information is relatively spared, but his performance on lexical-semantic tasks appears to be affected by the degree of

STM load inherent in the task. Assessment of his verbal short-term abilities is relevant to the hypothesis that he has a semantic access problem. WS's performance on digit and word span tasks indicated a very limited span (2-3 items) whether tested with a verbal response (repetition span) or a pointing response (pointing span). Although most individuals with aphasia have reduced spans a span of two is severe. Additionally, a two-item span in the pointing span task is consistent with a deficit in accessing semantics, as we have hypothesized so far. Performance on the pointing span task indicates difficulty in maintaining activation of verbal input in order to map the input onto semantic representations. This is more of a problem when items are part of a related set (digits). Additionally, although not noted in Table 16-1, when WS attempted to repeat more than two digits or words, he invariably produced the last two items of the sequence. That is, he was unable to report the primacy part of the sequence. This pattern has been associated with semantic access impairments (Martin & Saffran, 1997).

Overall Strengths and Weaknesses

Taking stock of WS's overall performance, the evidence indicates a semantic access problem rather than a loss or degradation of semantic knowledge. He can manage simple word-to-picture matching tasks fairly well, but does have some trouble when the pictures are of objects from the same semantic category. His scores on the synonymy judgment tasks are worse overall than on the word-to-picture matching tasks, but performance on these tasks also varies depending on the imageability of the words and their word class. The strongest evidence for this disorder being one of semantic access rather than one affecting semantic knowledge is his performance on the PPT test (Howard & Patterson, 1992). Overall, he found it easier to make these association judgments than the judgments of word meanings. It may be that this kind of judgment is easier, or it could be related to the paradigm that was used (choosing one of two items that is associated with a third item). What is most relevant is that his ability to make these judgments was near normal in the picture version and mildly depressed in the word version. This difference indicates that his knowledge of associations among concepts is preserved, but that there is some difficulty in linking that knowledge with words.

In summary, WS has a mild comprehension deficit that is exacerbated by context (discriminating among semantically related items) and task (those that increase working memory load). His production is fluent, but his anomia and attempts to retrieve words are disrupted by perseverations. The anomia is severe enough that his attempts to circumlocute are not informative. However, he is very responsive to phonemic and phrasal cuing, a pattern that is consistent with his intact phonological input processing.

Treatment of WS's Word Production Difficulty

WS's language profile, mapped onto a model of word processing is shown in Figure 16–2. An X marks a disruption of the bidirectional pathway that connects semantics with the lexical system.

The effects of such a lesion to this pathway will have greater consequences for production than comprehension. This is because the ability to map a word form in the lexical network to its semantic representation is facilitated by the structure of the comprehension task (e.g., having to choose from a limited set of pictures in a word-to-picture matching task) and by contextual clues to meaning in conversation. In contrast, in production, to produce a word, this connection must be strong enough to transmit a signal from a semantic representation with its corresponding word form that is competing with a large number of word forms that share some semantic features with the target word. This deficit does not disrupt the ability to discriminate words from nonwords in a lexical decision task or the ability to repeat a word. Also, presentation of a phonemic cue appears to boost the phonological form of the word sufficiently, such that the weak connection from semantics can effectively make contact.

WS demonstrated some ability to read concrete and highly imageable words fairly well. One part of the therapy program will take advantage of this ability. As described below, we will help WS develop a self-cuing system that uses written words and letters. To do this, he would have to be able to reliably read and understand common, concrete words. His performance on the Grammatical Class reading subtest of the PALPA (Kay, Lesser, & Coltheart, 1992) indicates that he can do this.

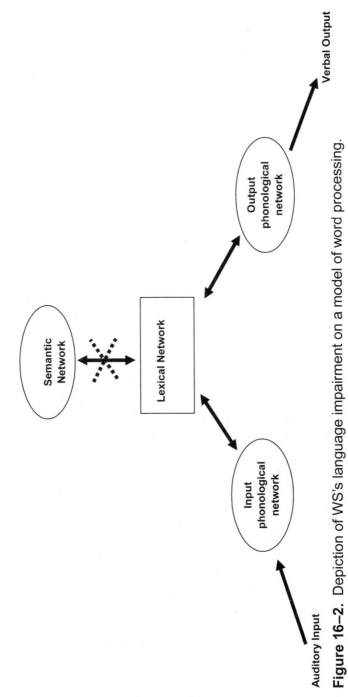

Figure 16–2. Depiction of WS's language impairment on a model of word processing.

Treatment Goals

The long-term goal will be to improve ability to retrieve words that are functionally important to WS in confrontation naming and in the context of spontaneously produced phrases and sentences. Two approaches will be used to improve WS's word retrieval, one that aims to improve word retrieval abilities using production priming treatment, and one that aims to enable WS to facilitate his retrieval of words, using a self-cuing training approach. Short-term goals are listed below in conjunction with the description of each method that will be used to achieve improved word retrieval ability.

Establishing Targets of Therapy for Both Production Priming and Self-Cuing Treatment

Items to be used in treatment will be developed as follows: Before treatment, WS will be administered a 200-item picture naming test twice with items from 10 semantic categories. Additionally, WS will identify words of interest to him that he cannot retrieve on a regular basis, including words or proper names related to activities of daily living and names of friends and relatives. From this large pool of words, we will identify 15 items that WS was unable to produce on either administration of the test and 15 items that he was able to produce correctly on one administration. These words will be the targets in both the production priming therapy and the self-cuing therapy. By using words that he sometimes produces correctly along with words he cannot produce independently at all, he will experience some success in treatment from the outset. This will help to alleviate any frustration during training.

Additionally, 30 cue words that WS *can* produce independently and which are functionally or personally valuable to him will be selected. These might come from the picture-naming test or he may decide to use words of his own choosing, as long as they are consistently produced correctly. These include words that begin with consonant phonemes in the phonetic alphabet (e.g., *b*oat, *c*at, *d*og, etc.). WS's self-cuing abilities will first be trained using consonant phoneme cue words and, in later stages of treatment, words beginning with vowels and consonant clusters will be addressed. Thus, these cue words will be used to train WS to self-cue his production of words that begin with the same consonant but that he cannot produce independently.

The procedures to be used in the production priming therapy and the self-cuing therapy are described below.

Design

A single-subject design strategy will be used during treatment, coupled with a pretest, pretreatment baseline, and post-treatment testing. The treatments will not be examined for their effectiveness separately. They are considered two parts of the overall treatment, one using direct drills to improve retrieval (the production priming) and the other to promote development of a functional strategy for managing word retrieval difficulty.

Treatment Sessions

For both treatments, sessions will begin with an assessment of WS's ability to produce the words he is currently working on. This will be in the form of a picture-naming test. The treatment part of the session will be divided into two parts. The production priming training will be conducted in the first part of the therapy session and this will be followed by explicit training in using the self-cuing strategy. WS will be encouraged to work on using the self-cuing strategy at home, and his wife will be informed of the words that he is working on. She will be instructed in the general approach to the self-cueing training and will be encouraged to help WS with his efforts to work on this at home.

Treatment Approach 1. Production Priming with Increasing Intervals Between Prime and Production

This method will be used to improve the ability to retrieve and maintain activation of a word's semantic and phonological representations in production. Massed repetition priming of words within a semantic class (i.e., training groups of semantically related words) provides some priming of the connections between the phonological form and semantic representations, but does so from a bottom-up direction (i.e., from phonology to semantics, which is opposite to the direction used in naming). This may not be as effective as a procedure that primes connections from semantics to the phonological form—in the same direction that is used in production (semantic → lexical phonological word form → phonological encoding). Martin, Fink, Renvall, and Laine (2006) modified the massed repetition priming portion of the task to become what they term "production" priming. Priming the production of a single word is accomplished by naming several different exemplars of a target word (e.g., five different exemplars of a chair). For example, for the target word "chair," the clinician would present five pictures of chairs, each in a different style. This method, termed production priming by Martin et al. (2006) will be used here.

An additional modification of this approach will be made in the following way: gradually, the interval between presentation of the prime and opportunity to independently name the pictured objects will be increased from 2 to 10 seconds. The rationale for this is that word retrieval depends on maintaining activation of semantic and phonological representations of words and that this ability is disturbed for WS. He can repeat words quite well, but after repeating a word he is able to produce it independently only for a very short time. It is hypothesized that practicing "holding onto" the word in short-term memory will help improve the strength of the connections between semantic and phonological representations of words.

In the original formulations of repetition and production priming, this method was combined with a context feature in which words being trained were related either semantically or phonologically or not at all. Research indicated that for individuals with semantic access disorders, training words within the same semantic category resulted in a good deal of interference during training (Martin, Fink, Renvall, & Laine, 2006). Although this interference (word substitutions from within the training set) ultimately did not interfere with short-term learning, the short-term learning effects were the same when the pictures being trained were unrelated. Given that WS has an access impairment, words within a training set (of 10 words, see below) will not include words that are semantically or phonologically related.

Production Priming: Goals and Specific Methods

Short-term goal: WS will be able to repeat a spoken word (from his core set of target words) and use it independently to name a corresponding picture presented after a specified interval (increasing from 2 seconds to 10 seconds).

Contextual Production Priming Procedure

Each item that is chosen for treatment will be paired with three additional exemplars of that item to be used in training. Thus, for the word *banana*, three different depictions (a black and white drawing, a photograph, or a color drawing) of a banana will be obtained. The items could be represented in different forms if the same name is used to denote each form. For example, pictures of several kinds of duck will be used as long as the picture does not elicit a specific name (e.g., mallard).

The production priming procedure will proceed in three stages of a hierarchy that moves the participant from naming with close dependence on a recent model of the word form (cued or self-generated) to naming independently of a recent model of the word form. Additionally, the time interval between hearing the stimulus and producing the name in response to a picture will gradually be increased.

Step 1: Blocked primed production. The four exemplars of the each item for training will be placed in front of WS. The therapist names each picture and WS identifies each one in turn. The first exemplar of the item to be trained (e.g., banana) is presented (the same picture that is used in baseline, test probes, and post-test). If WS cannot name the picture, he is given a phonemic cue or, if needed, a repetition cue to elicit the name once. Each exemplar of banana is shown one at a time for the subject to name (banana, banana, banana, banana) with just 2 seconds between presentations of each exemplar. This is repeated with 5 seconds between presentations of each exemplar and again with 10 seconds between presentations of each exemplar. Each of the five items that WS is working on (e.g., banana, newspaper, slippers, pencil, radio) will be trained in this way.

Step 2. Unblocked primed production—fixed order within sets. In this phase, the four exemplars of each name are divided into four sets each with one exemplar of each name being trained (e.g., four sets of exemplars of banana, newspaper, slippers, pencil, radio). Each set is presented for naming with 2 seconds intervening between presentations of each item in the set. The sequence of pictures stays the same for each set. Phonemic or repetition cues are provided if needed. The four sets are presented again with 5 seconds between presentation of each item within a set and a third time with 10 seconds between presentations of each item in the set.

Step 3. Unblocked primed production—random order within sets. In this phase, the four sets containing one exemplar of each name being trained (e.g., four sets of exemplars of banana, newspaper, slippers, pencil, radio) are presented again for naming, one set at a time. In this phase, the sequence of exemplars within a set is randomized from set to set. Thus, the first set could be banana, newspaper, slippers, pencil, radio and this would be followed by the second set of exemplars in a different order such as pencil, slippers, banana, radio, newspaper. Phonemic and repetition cues will be provided as needed. The interval between presentations of each item will be increased over three passages through the four sets of exemplars.

Treatment Approach 2: Development of Self-Cuing Strategies to Facilitate Word Retrieval (Nickels, 1992)

This method will be used to develop a functional strategy for WS to retrieve words. It involves identification of core words that can be retrieved and development of the ability to produce their initial sound, establishing a link between each cue word and words that begin with that sound but cannot be retrieved, and use of the cue to facilitate retrieval of that word. First these cue words will be written and paired with a picture. As WS becomes more familiar with his cue words, the picture cue will be faded out. Therapy will aim to help WS pick a cue word that begins with the same sound as a picture he is trying to name. He will be taught to isolate the initial consonant from the rest of his cue word and use that sound to cue the name of the picture. A concern here is that he will perseverate on the cue word and this will block production of the name of the picture. However, this will be minimized by the use of sets of semantically unrelated words, which generally provoke a minimum of perseverative responses (Martin, Roach, Brecher, & Lowery, 1998).

Self-Cuing Training: Goals and Specific Methods

Short-term goals:

1. WS will read words aloud and name their corresponding picture that will be used to develop his self-cuing strategy.
2. WS will be able to produce the initial sound of each cue word separately from the rest of the word.
3. WS will link a cue word and cue initial sound with one of the names of the pictures he is working on.
4. WS will learn to use the extracted cue initial sound to elicit the name of the picture he is working on.

Phase 1. Learning the Process of Using a Cue Word/Initial Sound to Self-Cue Retrieval of Another Word with the Same Initial Sound

From the 30 pictures that WS can name, 10 will be chosen that have the same initial sound as one of the words that he is working on via the production priming procedure. We will develop cue cards with the written word on one side and the picture of the word's referent on the opposite side. The initial letter in the written word will be underlined or colored red. Training will involve practice in identifying the initial letter and its corresponding sound. For example, if the cue word is baseball, the written word will be presented with the letter "b" underlined or in red. WS will say the word (or repeat it if he needs a model) and then will attempt to produce the initial sound. Once WS can produce the appropriate initial sound, the target picture to be named (e.g., banana) will be presented. WS will attempt to produce that name. If unsuccessful, the process will be repeated and examiner and WS will say the initial sound together to help him retrieve the word. Gradually, the use of the cue words will be reduced to cue letters written in isolation. A chart will be prepared for WS, consisting of all the initial phoneme cues.

Phase 2. Learning to Independently Identify the Appropriate Cue Card to Link with the Target Word that Begins with the Same Sound

In the first part of this training, the therapist identifies the target pictures-to-be-named that match each target cue word/letter/initial sound. A goal of therapy will be for WS to develop this ability without assistance from the therapist. That is, he will need to be able to look at a target picture-to-be-named and match it to the word in his cue inventory that begins with the same sound as the target word. Thus, the second part of his training will aim to improve his ability to match words that begin with the same initial sound.

This second phase will be carried out after Phase 1 described above aims to familiarize WS with the cuing process. This second phase is very challenging, as he must independently match cue words with pictures that share the same initial phoneme. This step could be difficult for WS because part of the disruption in this type of anomia is a difficulty in accessing the initial sounds of words. Provision of an initial phoneme cue is all that is needed to retrieve the word, but WS cannot do this himself. It is hoped that use of these written cue words will provide enough stimulation of the initial phoneme that he will be able to link it to the name of one of the pictures targeted in therapy.

Outcome Measures

Data Analysis: Acquisition, Maintenance, and Generalization

Progress will be tracked during training as measured by the proportion of correct responses on daily administration of the 30-item test used in baseline at the beginning of each treatment session. These data will be used to measure acquisition, maintenance, and any generalization from trained to untrained items. We will also administer the 300-item naming test following therapy and compare the proportions correct on this test pre- and post-therapy. McNemar tests of change will be used to determine overall improvements in naming.

Additionally, carryover of retrieval skills to extended speech will be measured by speech samples obtained before and after treatment. The Cinderella storytelling task and a picture description task will be used for this purpose. Our analyses of these samples will look for an increase in vocabulary, but also any improvements in sentence structure. Although WS is able to construct different sentence structures, he frequently does not complete sentences because of the word-finding difficulty. We anticipate that as more vocabulary is accessible to him, the sentences he produces will be more complete.

Summary of Treatment Plan

The treatment program outlined above focuses directly on improvement of the word retrieval difficulty that is the most prominent language deficit for WS. Two approaches are described, one which targets directly the word retrieval process (the contextual production priming with short-term memory stimulation) and the other aimed at developing a means for WS to self-cue retrieval of words in production. Thus, this program is focused on direct improvement of word retrieval abilities as well as management of the retrieval impairment via self-cuing. Although the focus is on the impairment, WS's overall well-being is addressed via fashioning the content of therapy (words that will be targeted in training) according to his everyday needs and interests. Additionally, his family's involvement is incorporated into the treatment plan.

References

Caplan, D. (1993, January). Toward a psycholinguistic approach to acquired neurogenic language disorders. *American Journal of Speech and Language Pathology,* pp. 56–83.

Crutch, S. J., & Warrington, E. K. (2005). Abstract and concrete concepts have structurally different representational frameworks. *Brain, 128,* 615–627.

Dunn, L., & Dunn, L. (1981). *Peabody Picture Vocabulary Test-Revised.* Circle Pines, MN: American Guidance Service.

Fink, R., Bowes, K., Grieb, T. & Martin, N. (in preparation). *Contextual production priming: Is it more effective than repetition priming?*

Gagnon, D. A., & Martin, N. (2002) Connectionist approaches to diagnosis, prognosis and remediation of acquired naming disorders, In. R. Daniloff (Ed.), *Connectionist approaches to clinical problems in speech and language.* Hillsdale, NJ: Erlbaum.

Hillis, A. E. (1991). Effects of separate treatments for distinct impairments within the naming process. In T. Prescott (Ed.), *Clinical aphasiology* (Vol. 19). San Diego, CA: College-Hill Press.

Howard, D., & Patterson, K. E. (1992). *The Pyramids and Palm Trees test.* Bury St. Edmunds: Thames Valley Test Company.

Kay, J., Lesser, R., & Coltheart, M. (1992). *PALPA: Psycholinguistic Assessments of language processing in aphasia.* Hove, UK: Lawrence Erlbaum.

Kohen, F. P., Kalinyak-Fliszar, M., & Martin, N. (2006, May). *The effect of memory load on measures of semantic knowledge.* Paper presented at the Clinical Aphasiology Conference; Ghent, Belgium.

Martin, N., & Ayala, J. (2004). Measurements of auditory-verbal STM in aphasia: Effects of task, item and word processing impairment. *Brain and Language, 89,* 464–483.

Martin, N., Fink, R., & Laine, M. (2004). Treatment of word retrieval with contextual priming. *Aphasiology, 18,* 457–471.

Martin, N., Fink, R., Laine, M., & Ayala, J. (2004). Immediate and short-term effects of contextual priming on word retrieval. *Aphasiology, 18,* 867–898.

Martin, N., Fink, R., Renvall, K., & Laine, M. (2006). Effectiveness of contextual repetition priming. Treatments for anomia depends on intact access to semantics. *Journal of International Neuropsychological Society, 12,* 1–14.

Martin, N., & Gupta, P. (2004). Exploring the relationship between word processing and verbal STM: Evidence from associations and dissociations. *Cognitive Neuropsychology, 21,* 213–228.

Martin, N., Roach, A., Brecher, A., & Lowery, J. (1998). Mechanisms underlying perseverations in aphasia. *Aphasiology, 12,* 319–333.

Martin, N., & Saffran, E. M. (1997). Language and auditory-verbal short-term memory impairments: Evidence for common underlying processes. *Cognitive Neuropsychology, 14*(5), 641–682.

Nickels, L., (1992). The autocue? Self-generated phonemic cues in the treatment of a disorder of reading and naming. *Cognitive Neuropsychology, 9,* 155–182.

Raymer, A. M., & Gonzalez Rothi, L. J. (2002). Clinical diagnosis and treatment of naming disorders. In A. E. Hillis (Ed.), *The handbook of adult language* disorders: Integrating cognitive neuropsychology, neurology and *rehabilitation.* New York: Psychology Press.

Renvall, K., Laine, M., Laakso, M., & Martin, N. (2003). Anomia rehabilitation with contextual priming: A case study. *Aphasiology, 17,* 305–308.

Roach, A., Schwartz, M. F., Martin, N., Grewal, R. S., & Brecher, A. (1996). The Philadelphia Naming Test: Scoring and rationale. *Clinical Aphasiology, 24,* 121–133.

Saffran, E. M., Schwartz, M. F., Linebarger, M. C., Martin, N., & Bochetto, P. (1987). *The Philadelphia Comprehension Battery.* Unpublished test battery.

17

Cognitive and Functional Interventions for Anomic Aphasia

Convergences and Divergences

Jacqueline Hinckley and Nadine Martin

In this section, we address ways in which the two treatment approaches prescribed for WS (i.e., cognitive, impairment-based, and functional treatment) are similar and how they are different. We discuss two interesting commonalities and one broad area of divergence.

One way in which the impairment-based and functional approaches described in this section converge is that both espouse a need to understand the full cognitive profile of the patient to appropriately plan and deliver treatment. Cognitive abilities, including attention, memory, and executive function, can impact language recovery. Thus, assessment of these skills is required, even though the degree of impairment varies across patients with aphasia. In the impairment-based approach, short-term working memory ability is particularly important to consider for devising treatment procedures and selecting appropriate treatment stimuli. This reflects recent considerations of the intimate ties between language function and other cognitive abilities that enable learning.

219

In the functional approach, use of strategies to accomplish communication requires clinical attention to the cognitive abilities that will support strategy learning and deployment. Cognitive mechanisms are explicitly addressed and specifically linked to selection of treatment goals, strategies, and methods for training of strategy use.

A second commonality across the impairment and functional approaches is training self-cuing strategies as part of intervention. The use of self-selected cues as a treatment procedure is shared by both approaches. Self-cuing is typically viewed as an impairment-based technique in the sense that it is usually discussed in the context of specific skill learning, such as naming. However, the partial control over treatment cues or stimuli afforded to the client is congruent with the shared decision-making aspect of the functional approach. Thus, self-cuing procedures can appeal to practitioners in both approaches.

There is one difference between the two approaches. Impairment-based treatment has been described as a "bottom-up" approach (Basso, 2003), in which language components, considered the "building blocks" of communication abilities, are targeted. The impairment-based approach "zooms in" on the impaired language structures or processes and provides direct intervention to improve them. The assumption is that treatment of specific aspects of language (e.g., naming) will have a broad, spreading effect across language and broader communication systems. The clinician uses the results of in-depth assessment to identify areas of language breakdown and language intervention targets that will bolster the entire language system. The contextual factors that affect the individual are not addressed directly, but are considered when treatment materials and activities, and contexts for generalization training are selected. Functional approaches have been described as "top-down" (Basso, 2003). They consider the individual's communication environment(s), and use these to determine ultimate treatment outcome. Assessment includes a thorough evaluation of the client's desires and contextual factors. This produces a large array of potential clinical directions or treatment choices. Treatment goals and procedures are then determined by shared decision-making with the client and by taking into consideration the contextual factors that will facilitate or interfere with achievement of these goals.

In recent decades, research in aphasia therapy has moved from asking broad, simple questions like "is treatment effective?" to more selective questions, such as "which treatment is best for which client to achieve which outcomes?" A simple comparison of a "bottom-up" approach to a "top-down" approach might lead to the idea that both approaches will arrive at the same point eventually—only the starting points differ. Of course, the picture is much more complex. Starting at different points and using different techniques may or may not lead to the same outcome. In the case of WS, outcome measures were described quite differently in the two approaches. But even when desired and measured outcomes are the same, the nature of the learning and the associated effects of treatment on other performances might be different across the two approaches.

More research is needed to address both general and specific outcomes of the two approaches to treatment.

Reference

Basso, A. (2003). *Aphasia and its therapy.* New York: Oxford University Press.

SECTION VI

18

A Case of Letter-by-Letter Reading

Linda J. Garcia

Case Description

LW is a 53-year-old right-handed man. He is a monolingual speaker of English and has had 11 years of formal education. Before his stroke, he was employed as an industrial plumber with an aeronautics firm. He is married and the father of three children; the youngest is 15 and lives at home, the two older children are both married and living in the area. He has one grandson, 2 years of age. Before the event, LW was an avid reader, reading trade magazines and enjoying adventure novels. LW and his wife have an active social life and a large network of friends. He played golf weekly and plans to return to the game as soon as medically feasible. He is active in the men's Bible study group at his church. LW reported that he wrote very little before the stroke—"mostly shopping lists and telephone messages." He commented that he has always been a poor speller.

Medical History

LW's initial symptom was the abrupt onset of a headache behind his left eye, and blurred vision. He recalled answering the phone, writing down a message, and not being able to read his own writing. LW was admitted to the hospital that day. A CT scan completed on admission showed a hemorrhagic infarct in the territory of the left posterior cerebral artery affecting the left posterior occipitotemporal region and extending into subadjacent white matter. Possible contributing factors to this stroke included mild hypertension and obesity. LW also has a history of mild sensorineural hearing loss.

At 4 days poststroke, visual field testing revealed that LW had a right hemianopia with greater density in the superior quadrant. This hemianopia completely resolved by 6 weeks poststroke.

Language Testing Data

Although LW was seen briefly for testing during his hospital stay, no formal language therapy was undertaken because no aphasia was noted at that time. However, he was seen in an outpatient speech-language clinic at 6 weeks poststroke complaining of his inability to read. At that time he was tested with the Western Aphasia Battery (WAB; Kertesz, 1982), the Boston Naming Test (Kaplan et al., 2001), portions of the Psycholinguistic Assessment of Language Performance in Aphasia (PALPA; Kay, Lesser, & Coltheart, 1992) and portions of the Gray Oral Reading Test-Revised (GORT; Form A; Wiederholt & Bryant, 2001). The test results are shown in Table 18–1 and summarized below.

On the WAB, LW achieved an Aphasia Quotient of 96.8 (within normal limits). His WAB picture description was complete, grammatically appropriate, and fluent. His Boston Naming Test Score was 58/60, also within normal limits. LW's reading problems were apparent on all reading subtests of the WAB except letter naming. Writing revealed spelling errors that were largely phonologically plausible. LW asserted that they were in line with premorbid spelling skills. This was confirmed by examination of some of LW's premorbid writing samples.

LW was administered the single word reading and spelling tests of the PALPA (i.e., subtests 29–36). Although the error rates were roughly 50% on all tasks, no word frequency, imagery, or part of speech effects were noted. LW was able to read pronounceable nonwords with fair accuracy. Regularity of spelling did not influence his accuracy. Word length effects were evident for seven-letter

Table 18–1. LW: Aphasia Test Scores

Test	Score	Test	Score
Western Aphasia Battery-Revised		**Psycholinguistic**	
Aphasia Quotient	97	**Assessments of Language**	
Information Content	10/10	**Processing in Aphasia**	
Fluency	10/10	**(PALPA)**	
Auditory Verbal		**Letter Length Reading**	
Comprehension		**PALPA 29**	
Yes/No questions	60/60	3 letters	5/6
Auditory Word 60/60		4 letters	4/6
Recognition		5 letters	1/6
Sequential Commands	80/80	6 letters	0/6
Repetition	82/100	*Syllable Length Reading*	
Naming		*PALPA 30*	
Object Naming	100/100	1 syllable	6/8
Word Fluency	18/20	2 syllable	4/8
Sentence Completion	10/10	3 syllable	1/8
Responsive Speech	10/10	*Imageability and Frequency*	
Reading		*Reading PALPA 31*	
Reading		High Imageability	20/40
Comprehension of		Low imageability	19/40
Sentences	38/40	High Frequency	21/40
Reading commands	2/20	Low Frequency	18/40
Written Word-Object		*Grammatical Class*	
Matching	3/6	*Reading PALPA 32*	
Written Word-Picture		Nouns	12/20
Matching	2/6	Adjectives	10/20
Spoken Word-Written		*Verbs*	9/20
Word Matching	1/6	Functors	10/20
Letter Discrimination	5/6	*Grammatical Class x*	
Letter naming	6/6	*Imageabilty*	
Writing		*Reading PALPA 33*	
Writing on Request	3/6	Nouns	11/20
Written Output	23/34	Functors	9/20
Writing to Dictation	6/10	*Lexical Morphology and*	
Dictated Letters and		*Reading PALPA 34*	
Numbers	38/40	Regular Inflection	9/15
Copying Words in		Derived	10/10
Sentences	22/22	Irregular Inflection	11/10
Boston Naming Test	58/60		

(continues)

Table 18–1. *(continued)*

Test	Score	Test	Score
Gray's Oral Reading Test-Revised (A)		***Spelling Sound Regularity and Reading PALPA 35***	
Comprehension	9/10	Regular Words	13/30
Reading speed	12.5 wpm[a]	Exception Words	14/30
		Nonword Reading PALPA 36	
		3-5 letters	18/18
		6 letters	3/6

[a]wpm = words per minute

words compared to shorter words. Letter naming was intact; however misnaming of letters was noted when LW was asked to read letters of single words.

LW's performance on Levels 1 through 6 of the GORT, Form A indicated that his reading comprehension was unimpaired (80–100% accuracy on all questions associated with the GORT-R passages). However, his mean oral reading rate was 12.5 words per minute, compared to adult normal rates of 150 to 200 wpm.

Additional Testing

Informal testing revealed that number reading, color naming, and visual memory for faces were intact.

Communication Goals

LW states that he would like to return to work in his former capacity, where minimal reading was required. He would also like to be able to read adventure novels and participate in reading activities relevant to Bible study class.

References

Kaplan, E., Goodglass, H., & Weintraub, S. (2001). *The Boston Naming Test* (2nd ed.). Baltimore: Lippincott, Williams and Wilkins.

Kay, J., Lesser, R., & Coltheart M. (1992). *Psycholinguistic Assessment of Language Performance in Aphasia* (PALPA). East Sussex, England: Lawrence Erlbaum.

Kertesz, A. (1982). *The Western Aphasia Battery.* New York: Grune & Stratton.

Wiederholt, J. L., & Bryant, B. R. (2001). *Gray Oral Reading Test* (4th ed.). San Antonio, TX: Harcourt Assessment Inc.

A Treatment Plan for a Letter-by-Letter Reader

Intervention from an Integrated Perspective

Linda J. Garcia

INTRODUCTION

This chapter addresses treatment for LW from both functional and impairment-based perspectives. From a functional perspective, LW's letter-by-letter reading disorder is interpreted in the context of its impact on his daily functioning. The issue here is that the reading disorder per se may or may not play a critical role in LW's life participation; other factors might be judged to be equally or more important. From an impairment perspective, the primary difficulty in daily functioning experienced by LW is tied to the language disorder itself. Hence, treating the reading disorder will improve those life participation activities which are dependent on this ability, thereby improving life participation.

The conceptual model that will be used for this therapy is called the disability creation model or DCP (Fougeyrollas, Cloutier, Bergeron, Côté, & St. Michel, 1999) and it is intimately related to the

International Classification of Functioning, Disability and Health or ICF (WHO, 2001). There are several fundamental principles on which this model has been designed, many of which are similar to the ICF. For a discussion of the differences between the DCP and the ICF, the reader is invited to consult Dr. Patrick Fougeyrollas' paper (2006) on the convergences and differences between the ICF and the DCP presented at the 12th Annual North American Collaborating Center Conference on ICF (http://www.icfconference.com/prog_pres.html).

A graphic representation of the DCP model is presented in Figure 19-1. *Life Habits* pertain to "a daily activity or a social role valued by the person or his sociocultural context according to his characteristics (age, sex, sociocultural identity, etc.), which ensures his survival and well-being in his society throughout his lifetime" (p. 131). The impact of LW's reading difficulty will be interpreted

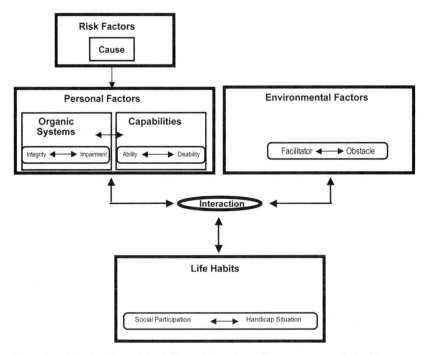

Figure 19–1. The Disability Creation Process model. (Reproduced with permission from Fougeyrollas et al., 1998.)

in the context of his life habits. An evaluation will, therefore, be required to identify those areas of life participation that are most disrupted by his reading disorder. *Personal Factors* in the model are considered intrinsic variables; whereas *Environmental Factors* are extrinsic. A personal factor can pertain to detail about the organic system or the individual's capabilities, for example, characteristics "such as age, sex, sociocultural identity, organic systems, capabilities, etc." (p. 34). Although the integrity of LW's organic systems (e.g., nature of his lesion) will be taken into consideration, the extent to which his capabilities are affected will be of greater concern inasmuch as they impact LW's life participation. Fougeyrollas et al. (1998) define *Capability* as "the intrinsic dimension of a person with regards to carrying out mental or physical activities, without taking environment into account" (p. 35). LW's reading difficulties fall into this category, as would any attentional or visual problems. The third important dimension (after *Life Habits* and *Personal Factors*) is the extrinsic dimension as expressed by the *Environmental Factors*. An environmental factor "is a physical or social dimension that determines a society's organization and context" (p. 35). Prior to commencing intervention, an assessment will be done of the perceived impact of these environmental factors on LW's communication. This model stresses the importance and relevance of considering the nature of the reading disorder as well as the role of environmental factors in influencing daily life activities and roles. The model depicts a theoretical representation of the interdependence of the three primary dimensions (Life Habits, Personal Factors, and Environmental Factors).

In order to plan for the intervention itself, another model, based on the DCP, will be used as a template for LW's intervention. The model (Figure 19-2) developed by Castelein, Noots-Villiers, et al. (1994) is the ESOPE (*Évaluation systémique des objectifs prioritaires en réadaptation* or Systemic evaluation of priority goals in rehabilitation). Taking a life participation approach to intervention, the model, which is a graphic representation of a clinical computer program, guides the therapeutic team through an analysis of the factors that contribute to the individual's life habits. The intervention plan designed for LW will be guided by this approach. The five principles on which the current therapy is based are described below.

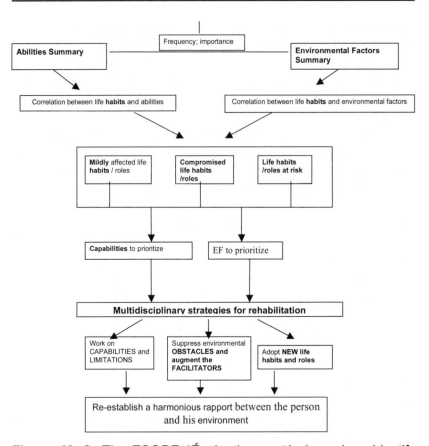

Figure 19–2. The ESOPE (*Évaluation systémique des objectifs prioritaires en réadaptation*—Systemic evaluation of priority goals in rehabilitation). (Adapted with permission from P. Castelein, P. Noots-Villers, et al., 1994.).

1. Similar Disorders, Different Impacts

The first principle on which this therapy is based is that the impact of a disorder such as a stroke is not identical across individuals. Applying this principle to LW suggests that, although we may be familiar with LW's symptoms of breakdown in reading and the underlying cognitive principles, the impact of these reading difficulties on his life is unique and should be treated as such. This assumes that understanding the reading disorder itself is only part of the solution. It is therefore not assumed that the impact of the reading disorder can be predicted from knowledge of the disorder alone.

2. Environmental Factors Contribute

The second principle on which this therapy plan will be based suggests that social and physical environmental factors can be the key to success. If LW is having difficulty participating in his life events and roles following stroke, then it is assumed that part of the problem is due to the context in which he functions. That is, some aspect of the social, physical, or organizational context is likely creating an obstacle or not facilitating his full life participation. Part of the intervention plan will be to identify the obstacles and eliminate them, identify the facilitators and encourage them, or create new facilitators.

3. Status Is Situational

The third principle that motivates this therapy design is that the current impact of LW's reading difficulties on life participation may not be permanent. This implies that the difficulties LW is currently having are not necessarily a reflection of how he will function later on in his life. Therapy, then, will focus on skills and contributing factors in the context of the present day life situation.

4. Functioning Is Not Discipline-Specific

The input of others (health professionals, colleagues, family) is crucial to understanding how, where, and when to intervene. Although intervention can focus on the reading disorder, the disorder must be taken into account in the larger functional life context. Hence, the input from other professionals is crucial.

5. Reduction of Impact Is the Goal

The fifth principle that guides the therapy is the realization that the ultimate outcome of intervention is to reduce the negative impact of the disorder on daily life. This will likely include improving LW's reading effectiveness. However, improved reading without diminished impact suggests that the goal has not been achieved.

In short, the first and foremost concern is that the reading treatment provided affects LW's life participation. This requires consideration of his reading abilities and functional limitations as well as the extrinsic or environmental factors related to them. Success is based on the interactions of both intrinsic and extrinsic elements. It is also assumed that as these factors change, so too will LW's outcomes.

Case Interpretation

The data available for LW (see Chapter 18) are focused on personal factors: both organic structures and capabilities. To summarize, the language test data are consistent with a diagnosis of a letter-by-letter reading disorder. There is also some information about LW's life goals and a bit of information about environmental factors. However, to design a specific therapy program, further evaluation of the latter two dimensions is necessary.

Additional Assessment

Life Habits Assessment

The first of the standardized tools that will be used is the Life-H scale (Fougeyrollas, Noreau, Dion, Lepage, Sévigny, & St. Michel, 1997; Figure 19–3). Items will be read to LW to determine his perceptions concerning his participation in various life habits. Each item (e.g., using services provided by a medical clinic, hospital, or rehabilitation center) in the Life-H will be evaluated using the following scoring categories:

- *Level of accomplishment:* LW will document his perceived level of accomplishment using the following rating scale: no difficulty, with difficulty, life habit is accomplished by proxy, life habit is not accomplished, or this item does not apply.
- *Type of assistance:* LW will indicate the level of assistance he needs to achieve each life habit: no assistance, adaptive device,

**Answer the following two questions.
(Check the appropriate boxes.)**

1 For each of the following life habits, indicate
A. How the person generally accomplishes it,
and
B. The type of assistance required to
accomplish it.

2 For each of the following life habits, indicate
the level of satisfaction with the way it is
accomplished.

Note: Keep in mind that answers should reflect the person's
usual way of carrying out his habits.

	Question 1		Question 2
	A Level of Accomplishment (Check only 1)	**B** Type of Assistance (Check 1 or more, as required)	Level of Satisfaction (Check only 1)
	No difficulty / With difficulty / Accomplished by a proxy / Not accomplished / Not applicable	No assistance / Assistive device / Adaptation / Human assistance	Very dissatisfied / Dissatisfied / More or less satisfied / Satisfied / Very satisfied	

Life habit	A	B	Q2	
Dressing and undressing the upper half of your body (clothing, accessories, including the choice of clothes)	○○○○○	○○○○	○○○○○	3.3.1
Dressing and undressing the lower half of your body (clothing, accessories, including the choice of clothes)	○○○○○	○○○○	○○○○○	3.3.2
Putting on, removing, and maintaining your assistive devices (orthotics, prosthetics, contact lenses, glasses, etc.)	○○○○○	○○○○	○○○○○	3.3.3
Taking care of your health (first aid, medication, following treatment instructions, etc.)	○○○○○	○○○○	○○○○○	3.4.1
Using services provided by a medical clinic, hospital or rehabilitation center.	○○○○○	○○○○	○○○○○	3.4.2

Communication

Life habit	A	B	Q2	
Communicating with another person at home or in the community (expressing needs, holding a conversation, etc.)	○○○○○	○○○○	○○○○○	4.1.1
Communicating with a group of people at home or in the community (expressing needs, holding a conversation, etc.)	○○○○○	○○○○	○○○○○	4.1.2
Written communication (writing a letter, message, etc.)	○○○○○	○○○○	○○○○○	4.2.1
Reading and understanding written information (newspapers, books, letters, signs, etc.) Note: If you use glasses to read, check Assistive devices	○○○○○	○○○○	○○○○○	4.2.2
Using a phone at home or at work	○○○○○	○○○○	○○○○○	4.3.1
Using a public or cell phone	○○○○○	○○○○	○○○○○	4.3.2
Using a computer	○○○○○	○○○○	○○○○○	4.3.3
Using a radio, television or sound system	○○○○○	○○○○	○○○○○	4.3.4

Housing

Life habit	A	B	Q2	
Choosing a home that suits your needs (house, apartment, group home)	○○○○○	○○○○	○○○○○	5.1

Figure 19–3. Items from the LIFE-H. (Reproduced with permission from Fougeyrollas et al., 1997.)

adaptation, and human assistance. From this information we will determine the perceived contribution of certain environmental factors in the realization of LW's life habits.

- *Level of satisfaction:* LW will identify his level of satisfaction with his abilities as they pertain to each item. Ratings for this level include a scale from very dissatisfied to very satisfied.

The items on the Life-H will then be summarized to give the therapeutic team an indication of those life habits which are most problematic for LW as well as the importance LW attaches to each item. Table 19-1 summarizes LW's perceived involvement in each of the global life habits in the DCP model.

From this assessment, several important life participation goals can be identified based on the frequency and value LW placed on them and based on the impact the reading disorder may have on his functioning. The following life participation goals can be identified as potential targets for therapy.

1. Driving to places outside of his regular environment (Item V in Table 19-1): Although there are several aspects of driving that impact this function, the impact of LW's reading difficulty on driving will need to be assessed. It is important to note that both reading speed and accuracy are necessary to improve functioning in this area.
2. Filling out financial forms (Item VI in Table 19-1): LW is not satisfied with his current situation of having financial forms read by his spouse. He would prefer to do this himself. Which aspect of this life participation activity is most difficult for LW needs to be determined. Complexity will be an important factor in this task. However, length of the reading passage may not be an issue for reading financial forms .
3. Participating in Bible class (Item VIII in Table 19-1): In terms of participating in community life, the possibility of unison reading and the impact of reading speed for the purposes of participating in Bible class should be addressed.
4. Going back to work (Item IX in Table 19-1): Returning to work may be problematic on many different levels, including LW's own adaptation to his new life goals. The possibility of improving reading to a level where LW would be able to read technical manuals needs to be explored. Factors to consider at this level include the size of the print and the complexity of the reading material. Technical manuals tend to be written in more complex language and be in smaller font thereby adding further obstacles to someone who is having difficulty deciphering written language. Speed is less of a factor than for other life participation roles. However, reading accuracy is very important. In the context of his work, LW must correctly

Table 19–1. Summary of LW's Perceived Performance on Each Life Habit

Life Habits	Elements Included	Level of Accomplishment	Value to LW	Comment
I. Nutrition (related to food consumption)	Diet, food preparation, meals	No major difficulties	Low	No reported impact of reading difficulty; not involved in meal preparation—spouse does it.
II. Fitness (related to the fitness of body and mind)	Rest, physical fitness, mental fitness	No major difficulties	Low	No reported impact of reading problem.
III. Personal Care (related to a person's physical well being)	Hygiene, excretory hygiene, dressing, health care	No major difficulties	High	No reported impact of reading problem. It is noted that LW can handle medication bottles.
IV. Housing (related to the individual's place of residence)	Lodging, home maintenance, use of furnishings and household appliances	No major difficulties	Middle	Most of the activities here are done by substitution (LW's spouse). LW is satisfied with this arrangement. There is therefore no need to intervene.

(continues)

Table 19-1. *(continued)*

Life Habits	Elements Included	Level of Accomplishment	Value to LW	Comment
V. Mobility (related or mobility over short or large distances with or without means of transportation)	Short distance mobility, transportation	Difficulties	High	Driving is a problem. LW needs to be able to drive to work and to Bible class and this is important to him. Sometimes he is called to drive outside the city and he may need to read street signs quickly. It is noted that we will need to explore the reasons for his driving problem. Is it related to a physical movement problem, to his inability to read street signs, or to another problem? We may need to refer as needed.
VI. Responsibility (related to taking up responsibilities)	Financial responsibilities, Civil responsibilities, Family responsibilities	Difficulties	High	There are financial difficulties due to LW's inability to work. LW also has the occasional government form to fill out. His wife currently takes care of all official forms. This is not satisfactory to LW and he would prefer to do them himself.

Life Habits	Elements Included	Level of Accomplishment	Value to LW	Comment
VII. Interpersonal Relationships (concerning relationships with others)	Sexual, Affective, and Social relationships	No major difficulties	High	LW's reading difficulties have minimal impact here. He is not involved with homework with his 15-year-old son. His reading is sufficient to not have an impact on his social life. He can handle social situations with friends and relatives with no or very minimal impact of reading (e.g., dinner, etc.).
VIII. Community Life (related to the activities of people within their community)	Community participation, spiritual life, and religious practice	Difficulties	High	LW needs to read to go to his Bible class, which is very important to him. The group reads and discusses Bible passages. There is a need to read in unison and at the same speed.
IX. Employment (related to the principal occupation of the adult individual; usually a paid occupation	Guidance, Job search, paid occupation, unpaid occupation	Difficulties	High	LW would like to return to work. He must read some technical information on products. He would prefer not to delegate this task to someone else.

(continues)

241

Table 19–1. (continued)

Life Habits	Elements Included	Level of Accomplishment	Value to LW	Comment
X. Recreation (related to recreational activities or others that are practiced during an individual's free time and within a pleasurable context)	Sports and games, arts and culture, and socio-recreational activities	Difficulties	High	Used to use the Internet. Now his spouse does this for him. This is not satisfactory. Would like to read adventure novels and trade magazines.

decipher the written material but has more time to do this than, say, deciphering road signs as he is driving.

5. Reading for pleasure (Item X in Table 19–1): LW enjoys reading adventure novels for pleasure. Accuracy and functional reading speed will be important.

6. Use of the Internet (Item X in Table 19–1): LW is currently unable to read information from the Internet. Speed may be less important than accuracy for this life participation goal. Environmental adjustments such as using the Accessibility options in Windows may be helpful.

It could be said then, that LW is living "situations" of handicap in each of these areas. Working with the assumption that priorities are best set by the individual who must live with the consequences (Parr, 2001), LW will be asked to rank these life participation events in order of priority. Because LW has no major verbal expressive problems, this should be done with relative ease with the clinician. From the case description, returning to work, being able to read novels, participating in Bible study class, and resuming driving would be priorities for him.

Assessment of Environmental Factors

Now that the important life participation goals have been identified and prioritized, additional information needs to be gathered regarding the influence of environmental factors. Applying the philosophy of the disability models, the situations of handicap that LW experiences in his life roles and activities would be influenced not only by his reading difficulties but also by the existence of supportive or interfering factors in his immediate physical and social environments. One of the objectives of intervention would be to suppress the environmental obstacles and/or encourage the use of environmental facilitators. To help the clinician identify these factors, a tool such as the Measure of the Quality of the Environment (MQE) (Fougeyrollas, Noreau, St Michel, & Boschen, 1999) could be used. The MQE asks the respondent to rate the influence of various environmental elements on a 5-point scale with "0" indicating no influence, –2 a significant obstacle, and a +2 indicating a strong facilitator. Although therapy aimed at the reading problem itself will likely bring success in reducing the situations of handicap mentioned previously, there is the possibility that these would further be diminished through the increased use of human help. For instance, with regard to filling out financial forms and the use of the Internet, LW has the help of his wife. It will be important to encourage his wife to continue in this facilitative role until he is able to do these tasks himself.

Summary Interpretation of Test Results

1. Summary of LW's personal communication goals (from case history)
   a. To return to work in his former capacity, where minimal reading is required.
   b. To be able to read adventure novels.
   c. To participate in reading activities relevant to Bible study class.
   d. To resume driving
2. Summary of other life habits and goals which might be at risk
   a. Using the Internet
   b. Filling out financial forms
3. Summary of functional limitations in reading (see Table 18–1 in Chapter 18, which describes the elements that one would include in the "Capabilities" box in Figure 19–1, this chapter)
   a. Auditory comprehension and verbal expressive skills within normal limits.
   b. Reading on all reading subtests of the WAB is impaired except for letter naming
   c. 50% error rates on the PALPA
   d. Word length effects are present on the PALPA
   e. Intact letter naming; misnaming when asked to read letters of single words on the PALPA
   f. Reading rate is slow (12.5 words per minute)
4. Summary of environmental factors
   a. LW's spouse is supportive for several life habits and roles including Internet use and filling out financial forms
   b. Reading novels is inadequate. No alterations are currently being brought to the text and no human assistance is sought at the present time for this task.
   c. Reading the Bible is inadequate. No alterations are currently being brought to the text and no human assistance is sought at the present time for this task.

   d. Street signs are presented too rapidly. No alterations are possible either in the form of text change or human help.

Treatment Goals

Based on this information and following the ESOPE model, multidisciplinary strategies for rehabilitation would focus on (a) improving the reading functions that are the most important for LW's life goals, (b) suppressing environmental obstacles and augmenting facilitators, and (c) adopting new life habits and roles. Therefore, in the case of LW. the following therapy goals are identified.

Strategies for Functional Limitations—Personal Factors

Two language-related goals are identified:

1. Improve reading speed: LW will need to improve his reading speed to adequate levels thereby allowing him to read novels, be involved in unison reading for Bible class, and read for work.
2. Improving reading accuracy for the same life goals.

Strategies for Environmental Factors

Several accommodations are possible to help LW return to his life participation goals. It was noted that individuals in his environment are instrumental in helping him return to his life activities and roles. For instance, his spouse was very supportive in several of these activities. However, language deficits resulting from stroke also affect spouses of stroke survivors (Sorin-Peters, 2003). In attempting to bring about change in the environmental factors, contact will be made with LW's spouse, coworkers, and Bible class colleagues to explore the impact of his language impairments on their life habits (especially in the case of his spouse) or on their interactions with him. These individuals will need support in the formal sense in terms of programs (e.g., spousal programs) or informally (e.g., information session). This support will then allow them to form a more supportive environment for LW. Other possibilities of environmental accommodations may be derived from reading material: Examples such as phrase-spaced paragraphs are given later in the chapter under the section "Therapy on Environmental Factors."

Strategies for Adopting New Life Habits

After analysis of the data, it may become apparent that LW must redefine new life roles. He may need to accept that certain life habits and roles may no longer be desirable or possible for him or he may decide, with some counseling, that the energy for changing a particular life habit is no longer worth the effort

Treatment(s)

The assumption for LW's therapy plan is that he is receiving care within a universal health care system similar to the one in Canada. The clinician may therefore work simultaneously on personal and environmental factors and subsequently explore the development of new life goals (Table 19–2). Outcome is based on success in identified life participation roles and habits.

From the analysis done above and to maximally improve LW's life participation in his life goals, he needs to improve both reading accuracy and reading speed. Reading speed is a priority in light of the fact that he has minimal reading comprehension difficulties. Several pieces of clinical data are important to design the therapy plan.

First, it appears from the case description and the results of aphasia testing, that LW's reading comprehension is unimpaired, suggesting that he is able, with time, to process lexically presented material. Hence, he does seem to have some implicit reading skills that can be useful for therapy. Second, LW's testing suggests that he has intact letter naming capabilities and can process other visual information. Hence, his reading difficulties are not due to a visual processing deficit per se. Remarkably his hemianopia has resolved, further diminishing the impact of visual deficits on his reading tasks. Third, LW is only 6 weeks postonset and therefore a candidate for restitutive therapy. Fourth, his deficit is indicative of a prelexical processing problem that impedes the access of visually processed information to lexical identification.

Table 19–2. Targets According to LW's Life Priorities

LW's Life Priority Goals	Targeted Personal Factors (Aptitudes)	Targeted Environmental Factors	Adopting New Life Habits?
Returning to work	• Reading accuracy • Motivation; personal importance of needing to work at this time; role definition	• Level of technical reading needed for his work. Identify tasks that require reading. • Time available for reading the technical material • Size of print as related to speed	• Start exploring with LW (in conjunction with other health professionals) the importance of returning to work at this time • Consideration of other new life participation options
Reading for pleasure	• Reading accuracy • Reading speed	• Types of novels that are available • Different input options for reading novels (e.g., auditory input)	• Role in discussion groups where novels are discussed. LW contributes to book club for persons with aphasia
Participating in Bible study class	• Unison reading • Reading speed • Motivation: Explore his perceptions of his role within Bible study group. Did he play a leadership role? Would he accept a less prominent role?	• Identify a partner in Bible study class to practice with LW • Reintegrate into group slowly as impairment therapy improves reading ability	

(continues)

247

Table 19–1. *(continued)*

LW's Life Priority Goals	Targeted Personal Factors (Aptitudes)	Targeted Environmental Factors	Adopting New Life Habits?
Driving to places outside of his regular environment	• Note: LW's primary difficulty in not being able to drive is likely related to physical/cognitive limitations. This must be explored in conjunction with the members of the rehabilitation team (e.g., cognitive demands placed on dual processing tasks such as reading and driving) • Provided the physical/cognitive aspects are adequate, work on speed and accuracy of reading. • Explore the importance of his role as driver. Would he consider being a passenger?	• Rapid presentation of road signs • Explore role of spouse in driving activities surrounding LW's life participation	• Explore new modes of transportation while driving improves.
Use of Internet	• Reading accuracy	• Explore role of spouse and teenage son in processing information for him • Explore aphasia-friendly Internet sites	
Filling out financial forms	• Reading accuracy	• Size of print • Exploring visual presentation of written material	• Explore possibility of relegating this task to spouse

The goal of therapy then is to (1) change the nature of his reading strategy from a letter-by-letter reading strategy as this is inadequate for his life goals and (2) improve the speed of reading word, sentence, and paragraph level material.

Treatment Design

Before commencing treatment, an unread text taken from a chosen novel will be used as baseline. Both accuracy and time data will be taken. This same novel passage will be used later to document improvement. LW will be accepted for a 10- to 12-week session block for weekly sessions. The first session will focus on 30 minutes of paragraph level reading using Multiple Oral Reading (MOR; Beeson, Magloire, & Robey, 2005) of fragmented texts. The second 30 minutes will be divided into 15 minutes of word-level therapy and 15 minutes of discussion regarding the impact of environmental factors. Additional sessions will be used when necessary to discuss with others in LW's environment or to visit these individuals in their context. Every month, probes will be taken to test LW's performance on previously unread novel passages. Criteria for moving to another passage of the novel will be improvement of reading speed to close to 80 to 100 words per minute. After 3 months, LW will be tested again using the baseline passage and re-evaluation of his participation in his life goals. Each treatment goal will be proposed to LW and he will be encouraged to ask questions regarding their rationale and expected benefits within the context of his life participation goals.

Impairment Level Therapy

Paragraph Level

As documented, LW's reading speed contributes significantly to his functional reading skills. The first treatment goal then will be to improve reading speed by developing therapy tasks that will increase LW's access to lexical word forms and circumventing letter-by-letter deciphering of lexical items.

As the intervention is focused primarily on the resulting impact of the reading disorder on everyday life, therapies which have proven useful for letter-by-letter readers which have documented changes at the connected speech level will be favored. One such therapy is the Multiple Oral Reading (MOR) technique. The technique, which is based on orally rereading passages, assumes that the semantic and syntactic constraints put on the text will facilitate access to the lexical form. It has been known for some time that reading single words in context is quicker than out of context (Biemiller, 1977-1978). Beeson and Insalaco (1998), Cherney (2004), and Beeson, Magloire, and Robey (2005) have shown improvements in reading using the MOR method. Although treatment programs for reading difficulties have typically focused on word level reading, this technique uses connected text. This method will therefore be useful for incorporating paragraph level text for improving reading speed.

Because LW's reading speed is very low (12 words per minute versus the normal 150–200 words per minute), we will incorporate a technique, which breaks down information into manageable pieces such as phrase-fragmented text. The parsing of the text in this fashion will make even more explicit the syntactic constraints. Inspired by the work of Jandreau and Bever (1992), Beeson and Insalaco (1998) used phrase-formatted text to treat a letter-by-letter reader. Jandreau and Bever (1992) used an algorithm called "Phrasetree" to assign phrase groupings to connected texts. The result of this process is that extra spaces are inserted to physically separate grammatical groupings. The following is a sentence taken from Fougeyrollas et al. (1999) regarding the DCP model. This is the text in a parsed format.

> The model "emphasizes the consideration of   environmental variables and supports   the collective project   of modifying them within the perspective that ensures the exercise of   human rights and equality (p. 18).

A series of passages from one of LW's chosen novels will be arranged using an adaptation of the phrase-spaced format proposed by Jandreau and Bever (1992). As per the multiple oral rereading task described by Beeson and Insalaco (1998) and Beeson et al. (2005), LW will be asked to read the first passage out loud repeatedly with the clinician correcting the errors as LW is reading. A list of some of the more troublesome words will be written and treated in the word-level therapy format. Reading rate will be progressively increased so as to attain the target. For practice, LW will be asked to read the target passage for 30 minutes each day. Once the target of 100 words per minute is attained, the phrase spacing will be removed and reading rates will be examined without the spacing. LW will also be invited to take part in an Aphasia book club fashioned along the lines of Elman's book club at the Aphasia Center of California (Elman & Bernstein-Ellis, 2006). He will have the opportunity to exchange the information that he has gathered through the reading of his novel with other individuals with aphasia, thereby maintaining the life participation goal of reading for pleasure.

Word Level

Beeson et al. (2005) have also noted that word length effects can remain despite the use of the MOR technique. In order to focus on the rapid recognition of single words, therapy will be modeled following the Sage, Hesketh, and Lambon Ralph (2005) study. Sage et al. used a letter-by-letter strategy and a word therapy strategy to treat a letter-by-letter reader. Although their participant showed improvement using both techniques, the letter strategy proved to be the least effective. Hence, he was more likely to maintain a letter-by-letter strategy following the letter-level therapy than the word-level therapy. Contrary to Sage et al.'s (2005) case, LW can identify letters; we will therefore use the word level therapy only. Fifteen minutes of each weekly therapy session will be used to treat single words. The material for these word lists will be the list of problem words identified during the paragraph level therapy and will be items related to the chosen novel. Therapy will begin with shorter words and progress to longer words. LW's family members (his wife and son) will be invited to help LW with this therapy 15 minutes a day. The target word will be read aloud letter by letter and then said aloud by the family member. LW will be invited to repeat the whole word. Scaling methods will include going from letter-by-letter reading to having chunks of letters appear at a time. If errors are made, LW will be invited to go to easier levels of reading until this is mastered. The words will be presented on a computer using the presentation effects option from PowerPoint. This option allows users to present letters individually and at varying speeds. Rather than present the letters themselves, we will opt to present the general shape of the word (see example in Figure 19-4). As the speed of presentation of the block forms is gradually increased to normal speed, LW will need to predict the rest of the word from the presentation of the first chunks of the word. For instance, in the example below, LW will use the visual shape of the word to predict which word it is. He will have the context of the phrase and the shape of the word to help him (see Figure 19-4). Errorless learning reading strategy will be used to make sure the strategy changes from his habitual letter-by-letter reading.

Examining Carryover

The effects of the above mentioned impairment-based therapy should show carryover to reading tasks involved during Bible class. However, because this life participation event involves unison reading we will alternate a 15-minute block of therapy every 2 weeks between a program called Oral Reading for Language in Aphasia (ORLA; Cherney, 2004) and work on environmental factors. For this exercise, excerpts from the next week's Bible class will be used in therapy. The ORLA program will also help in whole word recognition. The program, detailed in Cherney (2004), progressively brings the patient from listening to the therapist reading the passage and pointing out each word, to unison reading with the patient, while pointing to the words as he reads along. Rate can be progressively increased. The clinician then states a word that must be identified in the text. Speed with which the word is recognized in the text

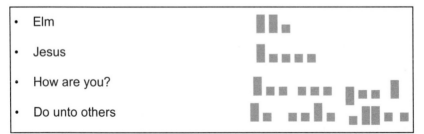

Figure 19–4. An example of reading stimuli used in LW's treatment.

can be increased. Finally, the patient reads the passage in unison with the therapist. During the regular therapy sessions, this will be done in unison with the clinician. During other moments in the week; the clinician will involve a partner from LW's Bible class.

Therapy on Environmental Factors

Every other week, the clinician will discuss with LW and individuals in his immediate environment about the environmental factors which are either impeding or improving involvement in life participation activities. Two areas have been identified for intervention. The first has to do with the formatting of the reading material he will be using in his life habits. The second has to do with the family, friends, and colleagues who are in some way connected to LW's life participation levels. For the text format, every other week the clinician will take stock of the possibilities for altering text information. Text can be prepared in phrase-spaced paragraphs for easier reading for all material other than that which is used for therapy. One such possibility is the Visual-Syntactic Text Formatting program for online reading of Internet information. As LW progresses, he will be introduced to an online parsing service on the Internet (http://www.liveink.com/LiveInkToGoReadingOnline.htm), which will help him parse out online text for easier reading (Walker, Schloss, Fletcher, Vogel, & Walker, 2005). The importance of adapting the reading material for individuals with aphasia has been documented by Brennan, Worrall, and McKenna (2005) and Rose, Worrall, and McKenna (2003). Using suggestions proposed in the Brennan et al. (2005) study, the therapy sessions will explore different ways of making the reading material LW needs to read into a more acceptable format. For instance, in addition to spacing text as mentioned before, the sheer amount of text might be reduced by adding pictures at strategic places.

In addition to working with an adaptation of the reading material, work on environmental factors will include discussions with LW's spouse, his son, his colleagues, and employer as well as with his Bible class colleagues. Preliminary discussions will take place early in the therapy plan to explore the impact the reading difficulty is having on LW's spouse and the extent to which she can be involved. The impact of the reading difficulty will be explored in terms of how it impacts LW's own life participation activities.

If needed, referral to other professionals in health care (e.g., a social worker) will be made to help LW's spouse identify with her new role as possible mediator between LW and his written environments. We will also work with LW's Bible class partners to identify a possible colleague who can help prepare the information for LW prior to class as well as help during the unison reading therapy.

Further family involvement is possible through LW's 15-year-old son with regard to driving. Lányi, Bacsa, Mátrai, Kosztyán, and Pataky (2004) have used computer software to help people with aphasia identify items in virtual worlds. Rose, Brooks, and Leadbetter (2004), at the same conference, reported on a virtual reality (VR) driving simulator assessment. The possibility of including rapidly presented words in a virtual setting such as a driving simulator would help LW use some of his impairment-based therapy strategies in simulated functional environments. Because of the innovative nature of VR therapies which are now available in many clinical practices in psychology (Rizzo, Buckwalter, van der Zaag, et al., 2000), involvement of LW's 15-year-old son is likely.

New Life Goals

As therapy on the impairment level and on the environmental factors continues, LW will also need to focus on his new roles and possible life goals. As needed, an additional therapy session will be added in conjunction with other health care team members. Working on his new identity is important for himself and for those closest to him (Shadden, 2005). These sessions will be aimed at helping LW define new goals and help him identify those previously identified goals he may now wish to let go. For instance, he may come to accept that his wife will now fill out most, if not all, government and financial forms. He may also come to reconsider his desire to return to work. This will be an ongoing process throughout therapy; as intrinsic and extrinsic factors change, so too may LW's life roles and goals.

Outcome Measures

According to the ESOPE model and as discussed previously in this chapter, the ultimate outcome is the "reestablishment of a harmonious rapport between the person and his environment" (see Figure 19-2) as expressed by life participation measures. Hence, outcome measures will be those that help evaluate the level of life participation as well as the relative contribution of the intrinsic and extrinsic factors. Life participation will be measured using a tool such as the Life-H. It is hoped that his levels of accomplishment will be rated higher for his chosen goals, with or without increased assistance as documented in the LIFE-H, under "type of assistance." These increased levels of accomplishment should also be reflected in his ratings of "Level of Satisfaction" before positive outcomes can be identified. This should be further documented in his perceptions of the environmental factors as facilitators or obstacles as measured by the MQE. The number of obstacles should diminish as the number of facilitators increase. More specifically, we may see more involvement of LW's son and colleagues and better quality of life for his wife. Measures of life participation and of the impact of environmental factors will also be taken 6 months postdischarge from therapy. At this time, we will be able to evaluate if LW has identified further life goals or is content with his current condition. The impact of environmental factors is important in establishing life participation levels but we will also wish to document changes in the impairment level functions as well. The GORT will be administered as well at 3 months and 6 months to document improvement in reading rate as will a timed word-reading accuracy test.

Summary

In summary, LW's treatment plan was developed primarily using disability models as a theoretical underpinning. Success and outcome is measured as a result of level of participation in life events, roles, and goals and intrinsic as well as extrinsic factors are seen to impact this level of participation. Therapy on the intrinsic factors focused on reading speed and accuracy and is couched within a functional framework based on life participation. Intervention focused on the extrinsic factors was judged to be as important a target as impairment-level therapy. In the spirit of giving LW ownership of his own progress, he would be consulted on all levels of therapy and explained the reasons for the recommendations by the therapist. The ultimate choice remains his as to which life goals to work on. Finally, the therapy would be offered in the context of an interprofessional rehabilitation team. The extent to which language impacts functions (e.g., driving) would be addressed by the speech-language pathologist; whereas other professionals would be able, using the ESOPE model, to visualize the therapeutic priorities from their perspectives as well as from LW's perspective.

This chapter attempts to illustrate how both the more traditional impairment-based therapies and more psychosocial approaches based on life participation goals can be integrated. In this era of outcome measurement and evidence-based practice, we are all made more and more cognizant of the impact of our interventions. An integrated approach offers not only the continued evidence that improvement in language skills can lead to changes in life participation, but also the certainty that, at least at an individual level, it can have life-changing effects. Furthermore, it ensures that work on social and physical environmental factors can contribute to improved quality of life for all who live with the effects of dyslexia/reading difficulty; thereby improving outcomes in life participation.

References

Beeson, P. M., & Insalaco, D. (1998). Acquired alexia; Lessons from successful treatment. *Journal of the International Neuropsychological Society, 4,* 621–635.

Beeson, P. M., Magloire, J. G., & Robey, R. R. (2005). Letter-by-letter reading: Natural recovery and response to treatment. *Behavioral Neurology, 16,* 191–202.

Biemiller, A. (1977–1978). Relationships between oral reading rates for letters, words, and simple text in the development of reading achievement. *Reading Research Quarterly. 13*(2), 223–253.

Brennan, A. D., Worrall, L. E., & McKenna, K. T. (2005). The relationship between specific features of aphasia—Friendly written material and comprehension of written material for people with aphasia: An exploratory study, *Aphasiology, 19*(8), 693–711.

Castelein, P., Noots-Villers, P., Buxant, P., & Spicher, C. (1994). Creation and testing of a "tool" for systemic assessment of brain damaged patients, *ICIDH and Environmental Factors Network Journal, 7,* 7–26.

Cherney, L. R. (2004). Aphasia, alexia and oral reading. *Topics in Stroke Rehabilitation, 11*(1), 22–36.

Elman, R., & Bernstein-Ellis, E. (2006, May/June). Aphasia book clubs: Making the connection. *Stroke Connection*, pp. 32–33.

Fougeyrollas, P. (2006, June). *Convergences and differences between ICF and DCP: The issue of environmental factors' influence in the construction of human functioning and disability.* Paper presented at the 12th Annual North American Collaborating Center Conference on ICF; Vancouver, BC.

Fougeyrollas, P., Cloutier, R., Bergeron, H., Côté, J., & St Michel, G. (1998). *The Quebec classification: Disability creation process.* Lac St. Charles, Quebec: .International Network on the Disability Creation Process.

Fougeyrollas, P., Noreau, L, Dion, S. A. Lepage, C. Sévigny, M., & St. Michel, G. (1997). *Life Habits (LIFE-H).* Lac St. Charles, Québec: International Network of the Disability Creation Process.

Fougeyrollas, P., Noreau, L., St Michel, G., & Boschen, K. (1999). *Measure of the Quality of the Environment, Version 2.0.* Lac St. Charles, Québec: International Network of the Disability Creation Process..

Jandreau, S., & Bever, T. (1992). Phrase-spaced formats improve comprehension in average readers, *Journal of Applied Psychology, 77*(2), 143–146.

Lányi, C. S., Bacsa, E., Mátrai, R., Kosztyán, Z., & Pataky, I. (2004, September). *Interactive rehabilitation software for treating patients with aphasia.* Presentation at the 5th International Conference on Disability, Virtual Reality and Associated Technology; Oxford, UK.

Parr, S. (2001). Psychological Aspects of Aphasia: Whose perspectives? *Folia Phoniatrica et Logopaedica, 53,* 266–288.

Rizzo, A.A., Buckwalter, J.G., van der Zaag, C., Neumann, U., Thiebaux, M., Chua, C., et al. (2000) Virtual environment applications in clinical neuropsychology. *Proceedings of the IEEE Virtual Reality 2000 Conference.* Los Alamitos, CA: IEEE Press.

Rose, F. D., Brooks, B. M., & Leadbetter, A. G. (2004, September). *Preliminary evaluation of a virtual reality-based driving assessment test.* Presentation at the 5th International Conference on Disability, Virtual Reality and Associated Technology; Oxford, UK.

Rose, T., Worrall, L., & McKenna, K. (2003). The effectiveness of aphasia-friendly principles for printed health education materials for people with aphasia following stroke. *Aphasiology, 17*(10), 947–963.

Sage, K., Hesketh, A., & Lambon Ralph, M. A. (2005). Using errorless learning to treat letter-by-letter reading: Contrasting word versus letter-based therapy. *Neuropsychological Rehabilitation, 15*(5), 619–642.

Shadden, B. B. (2005). Aphasia as identity theft: Theory and practice. *Aphasiology, 19* (3/4/5), 211–223.

Sorin-Peters, R. (2003). Viewing couples living with aphasia as adult learners: Implications for promoting quality of life, *Aphasiology, 17*(4), 405–416.

Walker, S., Schloss, P., Fletcher, C. R., Vogel, C. A. & Walker, R. C. (2005, May/June). Visual-syntactic text formatting: A new method to enhance online reading. *Reading Online, 8*(6). Available from: http://www. readingonline.org/articles/art_index.asp?HREF=r_walker/index.html.

World Health Organization. (2001). *International classification of functioning, disability and health (ICF)*. Geneva: Author.

SECTION VII

20

The State of Impairment- and Consequences-Based Approaches to Treatment for Aphasia

Final Commentary

Argye Hillis, Linda Worrall, and Cynthia K. Thompson

In this book we have presented examples of treatment programs from two "schools" of aphasia rehabilitation—one focusing on treatment of impairments and one focusing on treatment of the functional consequences of the impairment. What we as clinicians and researchers from the two schools learned most by coming together and discussing our distinct approaches to treatment is that we have more in common than we initially believed. We share an overarching goal to help people with aphasia function more effectively in their environments. We also agree that treatment should be made available to every person with aphasia. We share a belief that the person with aphasia should be actively involved in the therapy process, assisting with selection of treatment objectives and stimuli, and determining the frequency and duration of treatment.

We also adhere to similar principles of rehabilitation, including the well-known fact that treatment gains can continue many years after stroke, and the hypothesis that treatment is most effective if provided frequently. We even share many treatment methods. Where we diverge is in how we talk about our treatment, how and what we assess, how we formulate and prioritize our goals, and what we measure to evaluate the effectiveness of therapy. The chapters in this book provide illustrations of both the similarities and differences in the approaches to some common language deficits.

In our "consensus" meetings we agreed to make no judgments regarding what constitutes optimal aphasia rehabilitation. However, we dispelled many myths about the two approaches that have led to opposition. For instance, people in both schools believed that those in the other delivered only one type of treatment, their type. However, we learned that clinicians in the consequences school treat impairments, and those in the impairment school also seek to facilitate generalization to untreated stimuli, untreated tasks, and untreated situations to enhance everyday communication. As stated by Thompson in Chapter 1, "generalization to untrained language and to functional communication contexts is the gold standard of aphasia treatment, without it treatment may be deemed ineffective" (p. 10). Part of Martin's treatment included training a self-cuing strategy so that WS, her patient with anomic aphasia, could use it in everyday communication situations to help retrieve words. Howard proposed using a 'total communication' approach (Lawson & Fawcus, 1999) to facilitate functional communication. That is, treatment for his patient with very severe apraxia of speech and aphasia involved teaching GJ to engage all of his available resources (e.g., gesture, writing) to communicate, using the methods described by Davis and Wilcox in PACE (Promoting Aphasics' Communicative Effectiveness (PACE; Davis, 1980; Davis & Wilcox, 1981, 1985). Thompson explicitly stated functional goals for her agrammatic patient, TC, and infused methods for accomplishing them in her treatment: to improve (a) comprehension of real-time speech while listening in conversation, lectures, and other venues; (b) comprehension of written text in books, periodicals, and other material; (c) ability to express ideas and ask questions in group conversations, classrooms, and other settings; and (d) expression of ideas in writing.

Consequences-focused therapies should also seek to reduce impairment as part of intervention. There are numerous examples of this in the chapters of this book. For example, Garcia implements Multiple Oral Reading (Beeson, Magloire, & Robey, 2005) and word therapy for the client LW who is only 6 weeks postonset to improve reading speed so that LW can enjoy reading novels again. Hinckley describes how, for WS, lack of success in conversation skills training may require decomposition of the skills into smaller tasks that are practiced separately, but then rehearsed again as part of the larger task on conversation. Holland focuses on reading skills in her one-on-one treatment for MS, but the chosen words must have resonance in the client's daily life. Worrall offers her client attendance in a clinic within the same service that specializes in impairment-based treatment.

To highlight these difference and similarities, consider two studies in the literature of a profoundly aphasic patient, HG, who many years after major damage to most of her left hemisphere had fluent but meaningless speech. Hillis (1991, 1998) focused on treating two identified profound deficits—one involving the meanings of common words and one involving the pronunciation of common words. These two aspects of the lexicon were treated separately, using stimuli selected by HG to be important for her everyday living (clothes, foods, etc.). Hillis (1991) reported that HG could learn to distinguish related words, but the gains in semantic processing generalized only to words in the same categories as the treated words; they did not generalize to unrelated words. However, once she understood a word, she made fewer semantic errors on that word in all tasks, including conversation. In contrast, her ability to apply grapheme-phoneme conversion rules to pronounce words in oral reading generalized not only to other tasks but also to other unrelated words. That is, HG often accessed the orthographic but not the phonological representation of a word in a naming task, and then used grapheme-to-phoneme conversion to pronounce the word. However, this skill did not help her pronounce irregular words; she had to relearn the pronunciation of each irregular word individually. This learning required the therapist to spell the word the way it is pronounced (e.g., by spelling "scissors" as "sizzerz"), and then help HG to sound it out and blend the sounds, as HG could not repeat or compare her production to a spoken target. Nevertheless, with sufficient coaching and feedback, she could memorize the pronunciation of nearly any word. Although her improved pronunciation of irregular words was item specific, her improvement generalized across tasks (oral reading to oral naming) and across settings. It was reported, parenthetically, that HG accurately used the learned pronunciations in a restaurant setting.

A subsequent study (Hillis, 1998) focused on training HG both to semantically differentiate fabric names, and then to pronounce fabric names, to improve her performance at work as a stock person in a fabric store. What was measured in HG's impairment-based therapy were changes in HG's access to semantics and phonological representations of fabric names (impairment-focused), even though the patient's and therapist's long-term aim of therapy was to improve HG's success at work. In these two studies, the therapist measured "success" of therapy in terms of reduction of very specific impairments, and focused on these gains when describing therapy. Nevertheless, a great deal of thought and energy had gone into figuring out how to help HG function better in her environment. The therapist had learned, initially through gestures, drawing, and facial expressions, that HG lived with her 93-year-old grandfather (or great-grandfather, which never became clear), that she liked to design clothes, that she wanted to work (despite her profound aphasia and dense hemiplegia), and that she dreamed of going to Italy. The therapist visited her house on several occasions to determine what her communication needs were at home. She learned that the grandfather was nearly deaf and a bit demented, that HG did all of the housework despite her hemiplegia, and that neither could communicate by telephone until HG showed improvement in both semantics and assembling a phonological representation to say words aloud.

Once HG discovered she could learn to pronounce specific words that she could write (or copy from the newspaper, menu, etc.), she brought a list of 4 to 5 words to each therapy session, and learned to pronounce them. These words included everything from "good bye" to "Bacardi and Coke," and even "social democrat" (a phrase she copied from an article about Italy). Her learning to pronounce these words was never measured or "studied," although helping HG learn these pronunciations often required much of the therapy session. The therapist also helped secure HG a job through the state department of vocational rehabilitation, ensured her acquisition of an appropriate telecommunications (TTY in her case), and took her to "Little Italy" in Baltimore, as HG could not afford travel to Italy. Once again, these activities were not considered part of the "therapy," they were not documented or reported in the literature.

A therapist delivering treatment from a functional or consequences point of view might have gone about therapy in a similar way if they were providing therapy directly to HG. However, the measured gains would have been framed in terms of attainment of these personal goals, rather than her accuracy on particular language tasks. Functional therapy may have de-emphasized HG's deficits and had a greater focus on her environment by operationalizing the Americans with Disabilities Act and enabling her return to work through a supported return to work program and ensuring that her workplace was a place of equal opportunity. It may have also determined if telecommunications services for people with hearing or speech impairments (e.g., person-to-person relay systems) were appropriate to her. The therapist may have also enabled HG's travel to Italy by finding an "aphasia-friendly" travel agent or a support person willing to help HG with her travel plans. Perhaps the different approaches simply have a different emphasis in therapy. Therapists who focus on consequences also seek to improve component language skills and therapists who focus on language skills also seek to improve communication in everyday life, but their main focus differs.

One can surmise from the chapters in this book that the actual activities that took place during therapy were similar in the two approaches, although the descriptions of these activities and time spent on various activities were in some cases very different. Clinicians with a functional consequences approach devoted much of their chapters to describing how they would determine the individual's needs, goals, desires, and interests, with less emphasis on the impairment, in terms of testing to identify the locus of the impairment or explicating methods for treating it. Conversely, clinicians using the impairment approach focused on in-depth assessment of the impairment in order to determine underlying cognitive neuropsychological or neurolinguistic mechanisms, prescription of therapies to reduce these deficits, and measurement of performance on trained and untrained language, with less time spent in discussing the individual's relationships, goals, and barriers to achieving these goals. Although both types of clinician would "get the job done," there is much to be said for articulating what one actually does in treatment—whether it be the actual therapy tasks or how the individual's needs were determined. Foremost, teaching students how one can determine the functional consequences of impairment, as well as how to determine the nature of the impairments and how to address either type of problem will allow them to achieve a variety of laudable goals of therapy.

One important goal of the consequences approach is to change the environment. Impairment-focused treatment does not typically state objectives that involve changes in the environment. Nevertheless, clinicians providing this treatment often become involved in doing so, albeit it may not be an expressed goal of therapy. For example, impairment treatment will often provide advice to conversational partners about how to communicate with people with aphasia, and in some cases, direct spouse treatment may be implemented. Consequences-focused treatment would include changing the communication of the conversation partner, and consider it as the most important part of therapy. Direct intervention via conversational partner training would be provided because the conversational partner is viewed as the source of the communication disability for the person with aphasia. Whether or not change in the partner's communication ability is explicitly described as a component of therapy will reflect the clinician's approach. Hence, again, the difference may be one of emphasis in treatment. As Howard notes in his chapter, both approaches have the same end goals but have different means to achieve them.

Both approaches aim to restore the dignity of people with aphasia. Good clinicians are aware of the many variables that contribute to this and will spend time getting to know the person and what aspects of their lives require the most attention. These good clinicians will balance time spent in conversation, structured individual and group therapy activities, coaching, counseling, and socializing, depending on the person's immediate and long-term needs. In general, impairment-based treatment follows a medical model. The focus of intervention is on the aphasia itself, that is, the language impairment. The consequences approach is based on functional or social models and addresses the impact of the aphasia on the client's life from the client's perspective. What is clear from the chapters in this volume is that "healing" requires attention to both impairments and their functional consequences. Not surprisingly, helping individuals with aphasia requires both.

Bridging the gap between the two approaches must be a priority if aphasia rehabilitation is to succeed. Continuing to debate about which approach is better is not in the best interest of persons with aphasia or his or her family members, nor does this foster a positive professional image for our clients, students, or colleagues in related fields. However, continuing dialogues between experts in both approaches must proceed, and the case-based approach used in this book represents a first step toward a meeting of the minds. Indeed, the process has provided opportunity for proponents of each approach to share their techniques, which has fostered a better understanding of the similarities and differences between them. Clearly, this process has educated the authors. Aphasia therapists must be able to draw from a wide range of techniques to meet each individual's goals. Aphasiology is richer for having the two approaches.

This text has captured a moment in the history of aphasia rehabilitation. Until now, the two methods of impairment-focused and consequences-focused treatment have largely been discussed from an antagonistic perspective; however, we now have evidence that clinicians and researchers of both types embrace aspects of both. This has changed our attitudes and our thinking about what comprises optimal treatment. Indeed, it appears that both approaches can and should be used with persons with aphasia.

How can we foster and enhance this new attitude? There are two primary means. First, it is clear that if the two approaches are to be used, clinicians must be trained in both. The chapters in this book indicate that impairment-focused clinicians and researchers may be less knowledgeable about assessment and treatment tools used by consequence-focused clinicians. For example, Garcia discusses how to assess life habits and priorities; Worrall discusses Goal Attainment Scaling (Kiresuk & Sherman, 1968); Hinckley and Simmons-Mackie use the ICF checklist as a guideline for evaluating domains of activity and participation. Clearly, these and other measures were not used by the impairment-focused authors. Similarly, consequence-focused professionals may be less knowledgeable about how to evaluate language deficits within the context of cognitive neuropsychological and/or neurolinguistic models, to uncover the source of these deficits, and to treat them accordingly. Howard, Basso, and Martin discuss assessment within the context of models of lexical processing. Howard and Basso detail assessment of levels of word processing to ascertain the source of severe production and reading deficits, respectively. Martin also includes evaluation of working memory in order to understand the source of her client's naming difficulty. Thompson discusses in-depth assessment of morphosyntax to get at the root of sentence production and comprehension deficits.

Is it too much to expect that clinicians treating persons with aphasia be competent in all areas of assessment and treatment for aphasia? If we can agree that both "helping the patient to reclaim as much as possible of the underlying damaged capacity to process language [on the one hand and] treating the consequences of aphasia [on the other]" (Basso, Chapter 5, p. 63) are important, then we must endeavor to ensure that all aphasia clinicians are equipped to do this. The worth of the two approaches is not the issue; both must be instantiated to facilitate optimal recovery of language and communication. This does not preclude people with aphasia choosing one approach over another or aphasia therapists choosing to specialize and market their specialist skills, but it does require a mutual respect for and understanding of what each type of intervention provides and knowledge that our patients will benefit from them.

One question that often arises in open discussions of consequence-based approaches is: "Is treatment of psychosocial consequences of aphasia within the domain of speech and language pathology?" We suggest that it is. Aphasia is both a language and communication disorder. Treating both is necessary; therefore, clinicians must be trained to do both.

The second important mechanism for fostering convergence lies in continued research investigating the effects of both impairment- and consequence-based treatments. Our data, not our word, will engender confidence in the approaches that we take and will eliminate questions now, and in the future, about their value.

In summary, this book helps to clarify what is meant by impairment- and consequences-based intervention for aphasia and highlights areas in which the two approaches converge and where they diverge. The need for amalgamating the approaches is clear as is the need to continue to establish a strong research base supporting their efficacy. Both professionals and the clients that we treat will benefit from this meeting of the minds.

References

Beeson, P. M., Magloire, J. G., & Robey, R. R. (2005). Letter-by-letter reading: Natural recovery and response to treatment. *Behavioral Neurology, 16,* 191–202.

Davis, G. A. (1980). A critical look at PACE therapy. In R. Brookshire (Ed.), *Clinical Aphasiology Conference proceedings* (Vol. 1980). Minneapolis, MN: BRK.

Davis, G. A., & Wilcox, M. J. (1981). Incorporating parameters of natural conversation in aphasia treatment. In R. Chapey (Ed.), *Language intervention strategies in adult aphasia*. Baltimore: Williams.

Davis, G. A., & Wilcox, M. J. (1985). *Adult aphasia rehabilitation: Applied pragmatics*. Windsor, UK: NFER-Nelson.

Hillis, A. E. (1991). Effects of a separate treatments for distinct impairments within the naming process. In T. Prescott (Ed.), *Clinical aphasiology* (Vol. 19, pp. 255–265). Austin, TX: Pro-Ed.

Hillis, A. E. (1998).Treatment of naming disorders: New issues regarding old therapies. *Journal of the International Neuropsychological Society, 4,* 648–660.

Kiresuk, T. J., & Sherman, R. E. (1968). Goal attainment scaling: A general method of evaluating comprehensive community mental health programs. *Community Mental Health Journal, 4,* 443–453.

Lawson, R., & Fawcus, M. (1999). Increasing effective communication using a total communication approach. In S. Byng K. Swinburn, & C. Pound (Eds.), *The aphasia therapy file*. Hove, UK: Psychology Press.

Index

A

ACC (augmentative/alternative
    communication), 93–94,
    100, 116
  overview, 119–120
Accountability increases, 15–16
Adler Aphasia Center, 62
A-FROM (Living with Aphasia:
    Framework for Outcome
    Measurement), 12, 78–80
Agrammatism
  consequences-focused
      approach, 155–168
  impairment-based treatment,
      135–149
Agrammatism/nonfluent aphasia
  case description, 131–134,
      138–142
  consequences *versus*
      impairment approach,
      171–174
AIA (Aphasia Institute
    Assessment), 83, 85, 98
Anomic aphasia
  assessment, 200–208
  case study, 177–179, 184, 199–
      200

functional-social perspective,
    181–194
functional *versus* cognitive
    interventions, 219–221
and ICF (International
    Classification of
    Functioning, Disabilities
    and Health), 184, 186
lexical-phonological processing
    assessment, 206
lexical-semantic ability
    assessment, 204–206
outcome measures, 191–194,
    216–217
picture naming assessment, 203
production priming, 210–214
self-cuing, 210–211, 214–216
sentence comprehension
    assessment, 204–206
treatment, 188–191
verbal short-term memory
    assessment, 206–207
word production treatment, 208
word retrieval assessment, 203
AOS. *See* Apraxia of speech
*Aphasia, A Clinical and
    Psychological Study*
    (Weisenberg & McBride), 4–5

Aphasia Help?, 62
Aphasia Hope Foundation, 62, 97
Aphasia Institute, 62
Apraxia of speech (AOS)/aphasia
    ACC (augmentative/alternative
        communication), 91–92,
        98
    assessment examples, 78–86
    case interpretation, 78
    case study, 69–72
    functional-social intervention,
        75–101
    goals, treatment, 86–87
    treatment,
        functional-social perspective,
            87–97, 125–127
        impairment-based, 109–120,
            125–127
ASHA FACS (ASHA Functional
        Assessment of
        Communication Skills), 101
Assessment
    of activities, 82–85
    anomic aphasia, 200–208
    apraxia of speech (AOS)/aphasia
        examples, 78–86
    of environmental factors, 85
    and ICF (International
        Classification of
        Functioning, Disabilities
        and Health), 186–187
    of impairment, 82
    lexical-phonological processing,
        206
    lexical-semantic ability, 204–206
    life habits assessment, 236–243
    of multiple domains, 79–82
    neuropsychological evaluation,
        28–43
    of participation, 82–85
    picture naming, 203
    sentence comprehension, 204–
        206

subjective well-being, 86
verbal short-term memory,
    206–207
word retrieval, 203
AusTOMs (Australian Therapy
    Outcome Measures), 82, 98

B

BOSS CAPD (BOSS
    Communication -Associated
    Psychological Distress
    Scale), 86, 98
Broca's aphasia, 8
    and modern findings, 7

C

CADL (Communicative Abilities in
    Daily Living), 11
California Aphasia Center, 62
Case studies
    agrammatism/nonfluent aphasia,
        131–134, 138–142, 157–159
    anomic aphasia, 177–179, 184,
        199–200
    apraxia of speech/aphasia,
        69–72
    conversion mechanisms, 35–36
    fluent aphasia, 27–43, 36–40
    input buffers/lexicons, 34
    letter-by-letter reading, 225–228,
        236
    neuropsychological evaluation,
        28–29
    nonfluent aphasia/agrammatism,
        131–134, 138–142, 157–159
    output lexicons/buffers, 35
    semantic system, 34–35
CAT (Comprehensive Aphasia
    Test), 97–98
CILT (Constraint-Induced
    Language Therapy), 54

Cognitive neuropsychology, 8–9
Communicative Abilities in Daily
  Living (CADL), 11
*The Complexity Account of
  Treatment Efficacy,* 143
Connect, 62
Consequences-focused approach.
  See also Functional-social
  perspective; Treatment
  and accountability increases,
    15–16
  adult education, 165
  agrammatism, 155–168
  baselines, 162–164
  building on strengths, 49–50
  case study, fluent aphasia, 45–60
  and consumers, 16–18
  conversation initiation, 165
  and conversation therapy, 53
  disability models influence,
    12–15
  and disability movement, 16–18
  and families, 56–59
  fluent aphasia, 45–60
  and groups, 50–51, 164
  homework, 54–56
  and ICF, 12–15, 18
  versus impairment-based
    treatment, 18–19, 171–173,
    261–268
  with impairment-based
    treatment, 19–20
  individual treatment, 165–167
  information needed for, 46–47
  innovative/experimental
    approaches, 53–54
  one-on-one intervention, 51–54
  overview, 10–12
  personal interest incorporation,
    50
  practice, traditional, 52–53
  and psychosocial information,
    46–47

reading, 165–166
scripting, 54
and shared expertise, 47–49
and social model, 16–18
therapeutic assumptions, 47–50
therapy plan example, 50–56
CPS (Communicative Profiling
  System), 79

D

DCP (disability creation model),
  232–233, 238, 250. *See
  also* ESOPE (systemic
  evaluation of priority goals
  in rehabilitation)
"Dissconnection Syndromes
  in Animals and Man"
  (Geschwind), 6–7

E

ESOPE (systemic evaluation
  of priority goals in
  rehabilitation), 235–236,
  247, 256–257. *See also* DCP
  (disability creation model)
*Évaluation systémique des
  objectifs prioritaires en
  réadaption. See* ESOPE
  (systemic evaluation
  of priority goals in
  rehabilitation)

F

Families
  rehabilitation involvement, 56–57
  support for, 57–59
FCP (Functional Communication
  Profile), 11
Fluent aphasia
  case interpretation, 31–34
  case study, 27–43

Fluent aphasia *(continued)*
  conversion mechanisms, 35–36
  input buffers/lexicons, 34
  medical *versus* psychosocial
    treatment, 63–65
  neuropsychological evaluation,
    28–29
  outcome example, 40–42
  output lexicons/buffers, 35
  semantic system, 34–35
  treatment example, 31–43
Functional Communication Profile
  (FCP), 11
Functional-social perspective. *See
    also* Consequences-focused
    approach
  activities assessment, 82–85
  anomic aphasia, 181–194
  anomic aphasia treatment,
    188–191
  assessment examples, 79–86
  client identity treatment, 95–96
  emotional factors treatment,
    95–96
  environment treatment, 94–95
  and groups, 93–94
  impairment assessment, 82,
    184–187
  impairment treatment, 89–90,
    188–191
  multiple domain assessment,
    79–82
  multiple-domain treatment, 87–89
  outcome measures, 192–194
  participation assessment, 82–85
  participation treatment, 90–94
  subjective well-being
    assessment, 86

G

Geshwind, Norman, 6–7
Goal Attainment Scales, 98

H

Head, Henry, 4
Holland, Audrey, 11

I

ICF (International Classification
    of Functioning, Disabilities
    and Health), 11, 79, 87
  and anomic aphasia, 182, 184
  and aphasia, 15
  and assessment, 184–185
  conceptual framework, 12, 13
  consequences-focused
    approach, 12–15, 18
  versus DCP (disability creation
    model), 232
Impairment-based treatment
  agrammatism, 135–149
  *Aphasia, A Clinical and
    Psychological Study*
    (Weisenberg & McBride),
    4–5
  assessment, 200–208
  assessment, underlying deficit,
    111–114
  auditory comprehension speed,
    145–147
  cognitive neuropsychology, 8–9
  versus consequences-focused
    approach, 18–19, 171–173,
    261–268
  with consequences-focused
    approach, 19–20
  contemporary treatment
    overview, 7–8
  delivery of, 118–120
  "Dissconnection Syndromes
    in Animals and Man"
    (Geschwind), 6–7
  and functional language
    emergence, 137
  grammatical morphology, 148–150

history of, 4–9
and language access
    improvement, 136–137
Luria, A. R., 5–6
and modern neuroscientific
    findings, 7
neurolinguistics, 8, 142–159
outcome measures, 216–217
overview, 109–111, 120
post-World War II, 5–6
premises of, 9–10
and production, 144–145
psycholinguistic research, 8
reading comprehension speed,
    145–147
rehabilitation hospital-based
    history, 5
sentence comprehension,
    144–145
spoken output, 114–115
stimulation-facilitation methods,
    6–7
trace deletion hypothesis, 8
treatment efficacy, 9, 149–150
and verbs, 147–148
for word production, 208
written output, 116–117
Integrated treatment
design of, 249
and discipline specificity, 235
environmental factors, 235
environmental factors
    assessment, 243–244
environmental treatment, 245–
    246, 253–254
and impact on individuals,
    234–235
impairment-level therapy, 249–
    253
implementation, 245–255
letter-by-letter reading, 231–256
life habits assessment, 236–243
new habit building, 246

new life goals, 254
outcome measures, 254–256
overview, 231–234
reducing deficit impact, 235–236
situational status, 235
International Classification of
    Functioning, Disability
    and Health (ICF). *See* ICF
    (International Classification
    of Functioning, Disability
    and Health)
Internet resources, 62
Internet therapy, 55, 87, 93

L

Letter-by-letter reading
case study, 225–228, 236
environmental factors
    assessment, 243–244
environmental treatment, 245–
    246, 253–254
impairment-level therapy, 249–
    253
integrated treatment, 231–256
life habits assessment, 236–243
new habit building, 246
new life goals, 254
outcome measures, 254–256
treatment, 245–255
treatment design, 249
Living with Aphasia: Framework
    for Outcome Measurement
    (A-FROM), 12, 78–80
Luria, A. R., 5–6

M

McBride, Katharine, 4–5

N

National Aphasia Association, 62,
    97

Neurolinguistics, 8
Neuropsychological evaluation,
    28–30
New England Pantomime Test, 109
Nonfluent aphasia/agrammatism
    case description, 131–134,
        138–142
    impairment *versus*
        consequences approach,
        171–173

P

PACE (Promoting Aphasics'
    Communicative
    Effectiveness), 54, 119, 264
Post-World War II, 5–6
Psycholinguistics, 8

S

Sarno, Martha Taylor, 11
Schuell, Hildred, 6
SWLS (Satisfaction with Life
    Scale), 86
Systemic evaluation of priority
    goals in rehabilitation
    (ESOPE), 233–234, 245,
    254–255

T

Trace deletion hypothesis, 8
Treatment. *See also* Functional-
    social perspective;
    Impairment-based
    treatment; Integrated
    treatment
    and client identity, 95–96
    cognitive *versus* functional
        interventions, 219–221
    consequence-oriented, 45–60
        (*See also* Consequences-
        focused approach)

and conversation therapy, 53
delivery of, 118–120
emotional factors, 95–96
environment targeting, 94–95
and families, 56–59
fluent aphasia, 36–40, 45–60
functional *versus* cognitive
    interventions, 219–221
goals, 86–87
grapheme-to-phoneme
    conversion, 39–40
and groups, 50–51, 93–94, 98
homework, 54–56
impairment targeting, 89–90
individual, 165–167
innovative/experimental
    approaches, 53–54
integrated treatment, 245–255
letter-by-letter reading, 245–255
medical *versus* psychosocial
    approaches, 63–65
one-on-one intervention, 51–54
output buffers, 36–37
output lexicons, 37–39
participation targeting, 90–94
practice, traditional, 52–53
production priming, 210–214
self-cuing, 210–211, 214–216
sentences, 40
spoken output, 114–115
team management, 97
therapy plan example, 50–56
time management, 96–97
written output, 116–117

V

VASES (Visual Analogue Self-
    Esteem Scale), 86, 98

W

Weisenberg, Theodore, 4–5
Wepman, Joseph, 6
Wernicke's aphasia, 8

WHO (World Health Organization), 11, 12, 77, 85. *See also* ICF (International Classification of Functioning, Disabilities and Health (ICF)